PRAISE FOR *TENDING THE TREE OF LIFE*

It is difficult for me to overemphasize the significance of this excellent book for pastors, preachers, lay leaders and all who minister to people suffering reproductive loss. Speaking both from his own painful life experience and his expertise as a practical theologian, Richard Voelz boldly breaks the silence around the harm the church has done to people suffering from infertility, miscarriage, and other reproductive losses, calls us all to greater accountability for the way we interpret Biblical texts and theology in preaching and worship, and then posits a way forward that can lead to greater healing and wholeness for all. This book is as deeply thoughtful as it is practical, and is a first-rate resource for teachers of preaching and worship as well.

Leonora Tubbs Tisdale
Clement-Muehl Professor of Homiletics
Yale Divinity School

One of the great growing edges for the church – in the United States anyway – is a hesitancy to grapple with some of the very real issues of life. Divorce, addiction, infertility – these are things that often cause pastors to pause, trembling, as they search for words to bring some sort of light to bear on the heartache of such complex and painful issues. And, more often than not, this is simply because they do not have resources to assist them.

To that end, what Dr. Voelz has done with his *Tending the Tree of Life* is no small thing. Out of his own family's journey through the landscapes of infertility and adoption, he has managed to offer a tremendous gift – accessible, faithful, authentic study and suggestions for pastors and congregations so that they can better support and walk along beside the families in their contexts struggling through the same landscapes. Those of us who preach and pastor will be better at doing both thanks his work and witness.

Julie E. Richardson, M. Div.
Author of *AvailableHope: Parenting, Faith and a Terrifying World*,
Chalice Press, 2016

Tending the Tree of Life gives preachers and worship leaders an accessible framework for attending to reproductive loss and adoption in public practices of worship. If its claims are accepted, the text will expand narratives of faith and approaches to interpreting biblical texts in ways that support healing and well-being in our communities of faith. Voelz's personal vulnerability offers the reader their first point of entry into pages that demonstrate the greatest efforts of practical theology— namely, scholarship that has its beginning and ending in the everyday lived experiences of people of faith.

Lisa L. Thompson, PhD
Assistant Professor of Homiletics
Union Theological Seminary in the City of New York

TENDING THE TREE OF LIFE:

PREACHING AND WORSHIP THROUGH REPRODUCTIVE LOSS AND ADOPTION

ACADEMY OF PARISH CLERGY GUIDES TO PRACTICAL MINISTRY

Second Edition

RICHARD W. VOELZ

Energion Publications
Gonzalez, FL
2018

Electronic ISBNs:
Kindle: 978-1-63199-513-2
Google Play: 978-1-63199-514-9
iBooks: 978-1-63199-515-6
Adobe Digital Editions: 978-1-63199-516-3

Print:
ISBN10: 1-63199-512-X
ISBN13: 978-1-63199-512-5
Library of Congress Control Number: 2018935556

Energion Publications
P. O. Box 841
Gonzalez, FL 32560

energion.com
pubs@energion.com

Table of Contents

SERIES PREFACE

Clergy, having left Seminary, quickly discover that there is much about congregational ministry that they never learned in school. They have touched upon it in a practical ministry class or a preaching class, and an internship may have allowed a person to get their feet wet, but as important as this foundational education is, there is much that must be learned on the job. It is not until one spends actual time in congregational ministry that one's strengths and weaknesses are revealed. Continuing education is therefore a must. Having collegial relationships is also a must. Who else but other clergy truly understand the demands of this vocation? In addition to ongoing continuing education and collegial relationships, it is helpful to have access to books and articles authored by experienced clergy.

This series of books, the second to be sponsored by the Academy of Parish Clergy, is designed to provide clergy with resources written by practitioners—that is by people who have significant experience with ministry in local congregations. The authors of these books may have spent time teaching at seminaries or as denominational officials, but they also know what it means to serve congregations.

The Academy of Parish Clergy, the sponsor of this book series, was founded in the late 1960s. It emerged at a time when clergy began to see themselves as professionals – on par with physicians and attorneys. As such, they not only welcomed the status that comes with professional identity, but they also embraced the concept of professional standards and training. Not only were clergy to obtain graduate degrees, but they were to engage in ongoing continuing education. Following the lead of other professions, the founders of the Academy of parish Clergy saw this new organization as being the equivalent to the American Medical Association or the American Bar Association. By becoming a member of this organization, one would have access to a set of standards, a means of accountability outside denominational auspices, and have access to continuing education opportunities. These ideals remain in place to this day. The Academy stands as a beacon to clergy looking for support and accountability in an age when even the religious vocation is no longer held in high esteem.

In 2012, the Academy launched its first book series in partnership with Energion Publications. This series, entitled *Conversations in Ministry*, fits closely with an important part of the mission of the Academy—encouraging clergy to gather in groups to support one another and hold each other accountable in their local ministry settings. The books in this first series are brief (under 100 pages), making them useful for igniting conversation.

This second series, *Guides to Practical Ministry*, features longer books. Like the first series these books are written by clergy for clergy. They can be used by groups, but because they are lengthier in scope, they can go into greater depth than the books found the first series. Books in this series will cover issues like writing sermons, interim ministry, self-care, clergy ethics, administrative tasks, the use of social media, worship leadership. In the case of this book, the focus is preaching in the context of reproductive loss and adoption.

On behalf of the Academy of Parish Clergy, the series' editorial team, and the publisher, I pray that the books in this series will be a blessing to all who read them and to all who receive them through the ministry of these readers.

Robert D. Cornwall, FAPC
General Editor

Acknowledgements

When I entered graduate studies in homiletics and liturgics, I had no idea that this would be one of the areas in which I would conduct research and write. In fact, much of my research for this book has come through my own personal experiences brought together with my graduate training. For that, I give much credit to the faculty in Homiletics and Liturgics during my time at Vanderbilt University: John S. McClure, Brad R. Braxton, Ted A. Smith, Robin M. Jensen, and the late Dale P. Andrews. Each supplied me with resources to engage in homiletic and liturgical reflection on this very personal topic. Seven days after I became "Doctor Voelz," I became "Dad." Their support was invaluable to me as I negotiated both of those identities.

I had a very supportive group of colleagues throughout my graduate studies who also encouraged me as I wrote this book post-graduation. Amy Peed McCullough, Katy Rigler, Noel Schoonmaker, Mark Shivers, Alex Tracy, Joshua Villines as well as Gerald Liu, Brandon McCormack, and Lisa Thompson have all made me better at what I do. I should also acknowledge my colleagues in the Academy of Homiletics who have encouraged this work in conversations along the way.

The people of Central Christian Church (Disciples of Christ) in Springfield, Tennessee provided a tremendous pastorate experience as I finished my doctoral work and as we (almost simultaneously) received our daughter into our home. Their love and encouragement, as well as the stories they shared of adoption in such a small congregational setting was truly an encounter with the Divine. Johns Creek Christian Church (Disciples of Christ) in Johns Creek, Georgia where I also served as senior minister, encouraged this project, allowing their minister opportunities to disappear for dedicated writing times and checking in from time-to-time on the progress of the book. What a joy it was to minister with them in the journey of being church.

I have had the opportunity to teach through this book with students at Union Presbyterian Seminary in Richmond, VA where I serve as Assistant Professor of Preaching & Worship. In a course I co-taught with John T. Carroll called "Children and Youth in the Bible and in the Worship of the Church," student interaction was extremely generative. I hope that others will find it as such.

Our adoption would not have taken place without the superlative staff at Miriam's Promise, our agency in Nashville, Tennessee. I have a difficult time imagining a better group of people to help facilitate the adoption process. They provided us training and support, treated our daughter's birth family with utmost respect, waited for hours with us in the hospital, and helped us finalize our adoption. The care and professionalism with which they treated us and the other waiting families in our "cohort" was tremendous. It is my deepest hope that they will be honored by this book.

My original editor, Todd Edmondson, believed in the importance of this project and was a patient guide throughout the process with Shook Foil Books, where this book first appeared in a digital edition. As it comes into another publishing house, I thank Bob Cornwall who approached me about bringing it to print, The Academy of Parish Clergy, as well as Henry and Jody Neufeld of Energion Publications.

My friend and artist, Nathan D. Pelton, designed the art piece that is the cover art for the book. It perfectly captures the spirit of the book and I thank him for his beautiful contribution.

Finally, and most importantly, I must thank my wife Meredith for her support in my writing this book. She has given permission to put parts of our personal lives on display, with the hopes that it will be helpful for those charged with the spiritual care of families who experience reproductive loss and adoption. Without her willingness and her belief in the kind of work I do, this project would not see the light of day. She has been just the kind of wonderful mother to our daughter I thought she would be.

– *Richard Voelz*

INTRODUCTION

MY STORY

In the Spring of 2006, my wife and I decided that it was time for us to begin the process of building our family. Like many young professional couples, we had put off having children as we made our way through seminary and graduate school, began careers, discovered what it meant to be married, and attempted to gain some sense of financial stability. Having been admitted to the PhD program in Homiletics and Liturgics and Vanderbilt University in that spring, we believed this was the time for us to finally do what we had been putting off.

Of course, we assumed that having biological children would be a relatively easy process. Many of our similarly-aged friends seemed to be having no problem succeeding in this area of life and as healthy young adults we had no reason to believe we would encounter any difficulty. Time passed with no success. Charting temperatures and ovulation cycles yielded no results. After a year, we began the process of fertility testing. I was the first to enter those cold doctors' offices for tests and diagnoses. The experience was life-changing, to say the least. At one doctor's office, I was given a bracelet to wear in the waiting room with a number that corresponded to my file. It felt like a flashing neon sign around my wrist as I waited to be called like one among a herd of animals. The attending nurse would check to make sure that this number matched the file as I was called back for consultation and testing. Later, we would switch doctors for a more personal experience. My spouse certainly had the more invasive experience, with frequent blood tests and sonograms to determine various types of levels and counts.

Ultimately it was determined that we were largely in the "unexplained infertility" category. We did not know people who had gone through this, and it is not something that couples usually broadcast (at least we did not), so we had little wise counsel from which to make our decisions. We resolved to go through as much and as many fertility treatments as we could afford and until we felt like we had exhausted our options of having biological children. That was an indefinite line, but we thought we would know that at some point we would reach a place where we could either achieve what we wanted or easily be able to say, "Enough." We went through three different types of treatments that escalated in cost, invasiveness, and preparation, including the most invasive, IVF (in vitro fertilization), all to no avail. After our failed IVF experience, we agreed that we had reached our line.

The treatments were grueling processes, which included giving injections to my wife intended to prepare her body so that the doctor could time the procedures precisely for the best chance at conception and implantation. Our IVF process yielded two embryos, neither of which would be classified as strong candidates for continued growth or implantation. The cycles of hope and disappointment were nerve-wracking, with weeks of preparation, hope, and waiting, each ending in disappointment.

In the back of our minds, we had thought about adoption and had even spoken about it, but it did not merit serious discussion until our final fertility treatment (IVF) was unsuccessful. We grieved the end of the pursuit of biological children as a loss and tried to make sense of the ways that our bodies had betrayed us. We read books. We talked. We breathed deeply and prayed. We bought a new flat-screen television (admittedly, this was not the best way of coping). We began studying about adoption. But we did not have many places to turn that enabled us to process what we were going through or where we felt understood or safe. And of chief importance, we certainly did not feel as if our spiritual needs were being met in our communities of faith.

Throughout this time, I was a doctoral student in preaching and worship and someone who faithfully occupied the pew every week. My wife and I tried to find a faith community of which we could be a part. Everywhere we visited we were asked almost immediately, "So, do you have kids?" We quickly realized that "young family with children" is a hot commodity for congregations, as our single friends often suggest is the case.

As I heard the stories of Abraham and Sarah conceiving during one Ordinary Time lectionary cycle and subsequently journeyed through Advent, I heard again the stories of the conceptions of John the Baptist and Jesus, only this time through a new set of interpretive lenses. In doing so, I became increasingly frustrated in my faith. Nowhere were these stories related to the experiences I was having. The difficulties of conception were not acknowledged, nor were the real losses of fertility loss or the miscarriages my friends were experiencing. Miracle births were treated as acceptable and understandable occurrences built into the consciousness of faith.

As we made the transition to becoming a waiting family in the adoption process, I likewise never heard a word about adoption in preaching or worship. We worked with a wonderful adoption agency whose counselors educated us, advised us, encouraged us, and provided the best environment I could possibly imagine to prepare us for the journey on which adoption would take us. We chose to adopt domestically (which, to be clear, is no better or worse than any other kind of adoption; it was just the right decision for how we wanted to build our family) and completed the requisite mountains of paperwork prior to our approval.

During this time I also took a located pastorate as I finished my dissertation. The initial greeting I wrote to my new congregation was about Advent and waiting for children of promise:

> As we move through Advent this year, we are certainly living into the major themes of Advent—"waiting," "expectation," and "anticipation" —in so many ways. We are, of course, awaiting the celebration of the birth of Jesus. Each year we are reminded of God's great love demonstrated through God's desire to take on flesh and dwell among us. It is difficult to wait on celebrating that—to truly live in expectation when everything surrounding us calls us to hurry toward that manger. And yet, we try to wait. We also know a bit about waiting

for a child. Meredith and I are in the process of adoption and are currently waiting on a placement. Advent is a reminder to us that we do not do our waiting in vain. Our waiting is always in hopeful anticipation of something great—something greater than we can imagine as God works in this world. And finally, we also know about waiting for a relationship. Jesus came into this world as a living sign that all people can live in relationship with God and in peace with one other. Confident in the promise of that kind of relationship, we wait this Advent eager to begin our relationships with [the congregation] and with each of you."

After a period of completing agency training, home visits by state-approved social workers, and again, much waiting, as I sat in a Wednesday morning meeting for teaching assistants for Vanderbilt's introductory preaching class, I was surprised with a phone call that a baby girl had been born on Monday. The birthmother of that child had chosen us after making the decision that she would not parent the baby. We had nothing ready in our house to receive a child. We had painted the room that was still functioning as a guest room and we had a crib in a box in the garage, but that was as ready as we were. Beyond that, we had nothing. My wife just happened to be a plane ride away on a spring break vacation in another state. After rushing her back the day of the phone call and hurriedly acquiring some essentials, we set out the next day to a hospital about two hours from our home to meet the birthmother and pick up our child. In 24 hours (and a week to the day after I had defended my dissertation), we became parents. Our daughter slept her first few nights in a blanketed laundry basket. We told only a few people until the period for the birthmother to waive her rights was legally over. Much of her story is hers to tell when and if she chooses to do so. I'm glad to say that at the time this book is republished, our daughter is happy, healthy, and truly a joy at seven years old.

REPRODUCTIVE LOSS, ADOPTION, AND WRITING FROM A PLACE

I know many other couples whose journeys through various types of reproductive loss have been met with equal parts disappointment and success. And I know others who have journeyed through adoption with struggle and joy. In talking with many of them, I understand that some faith communities and congregations are doing a good job of addressing the spiritual concerns these life experiences bring. Mostly I think this happens in congregations where there are sufficient numbers of young adults who happen to be experiencing reproductive loss or where adoptions occur among congregants with some regularity. And this happens through relationships formed in community and excellent pastoral care. I believe that these communities of faith are special, and I am thankful for the ways that they have provided care for their congregants, but I believe that they are in the minority (particularly among so-called mainline denominational/progressive congregations, which is my primary orientation).

At the outset, it will be helpful for me to define a major term that I use both in the subtitle of the book and throughout the book. I will often refer to the term "reproductive loss." I use this as a blanket term describing experiences of infertility (in all its varying degrees) and loss of fertility, miscarriage, stillbirth, and other forms of pregnancy loss. Serene Jones says

> In clinical terms, infertility describes a biological condition in which conception cannot take place (although it is often expanded to include biological conditions in which a fertilized egg cannot be sustained in utero for any number of reasons, including genetic ones); a miscarriage (often referred to as a spontaneous abortion) is the loss of a pregnancy after conception but before twenty-four weeks; stillbirth is the loss of a pregnancy any time from twenty-four weeks to term in which the fetus dies in utero or immediately following delivery (in many such cases, the fetus must be "delivered" either by Cesarean or vaginal birth, and hence the term "stillbirth")...I

am interested in looking at the experience of women who desire to have biological children, who are biologically unable to do so, and who experience this bodily inability as failure, a desire thwarted, a loss of a potential child they hoped for and expected.[1]

Certainly no one term can do justice to the entire range of individuals' experiences, but the word "loss" is important. Even though my wife and I were not able to conceive, acknowledging the truth of that came as a loss: a loss of hope, a loss of dreams, a loss of expectations, and a loss of control over one's body. Others will likely express different perceptions of loss, but each kind of loss is real. Pastors who are privileged to minister in these situations will do well to recognize these different kinds of loss.

I should also differentiate between some other terms with which uninitiated readers might be unfamiliar: biological children, birthparent/biological parent, adoptive parent, etc. These will unfold throughout the course of the book.

This book admittedly grows out of my own experiences and reflections on those experiences. Though I try to be inclusive on a number of issues regarding reproductive loss and adoption, I do not claim to speak with authority about the experiences of all men or women, or those pursuing reproductive medicine and adoptive families. Each situation is different. My wife and I never conceived and thus we did not grapple with the loss of miscarriage or pregnancy loss, though I try my best to be sensitive of those who have.

Additionally, I am a male writing about reproductive loss and adoption as someone with particular experiences in those areas. This complexity is not lost on me. I understand that women will almost certainly experience these situations in markedly different ways than I did/do as a male. I do not see this partiality as a limitation, nor do I fear offending feminist sensibilities. I do not try to speak in the place of female experiences. Still, I invite readers

---

1   Serene Jones, *Trauma and Grace: Theology in a Ruptured World* (Louisville, KY: Westminster John Knox Press, 2009), 130. As a male, I extend my treatment to men as well.

to use what I write here as a jumping off point for their reflections in the particularity of their experiences, noting the similarities and differences along the way.

Furthermore, I write as a practical theologian in the field of homiletics and liturgics. This is not a constructive theology of reproductive loss and adoption, though I hope to faithfully use the resources within the field for an integrative, practical theological work. My main goals are to improve the conditions of, and provide resources for, preaching and worship as congregational experiences as they relate to reproductive loss and adoption.

As my wife and I began to open up in ecclesial settings, personal relationships, and on social media about reproductive loss and adoption, we found that we were in the company of a great number of people of faith that either had or were having experiences with either of these subjects or both, both young and old. I am grateful for the honesty with which they shared their experiences with me and I hope this book honors their contributions to my reflection on this subject.

Many readers might recognize that the title line of this book emerges from Proverbs 13:12: "Hope deferred makes the heart sick, but a desire fulfilled is a tree of life." Although I do not believe that I speak for the experiences of all people, as I say above, I do believe that anyone who has experienced the heartaches of reproductive loss and the cycles of hope/despair associated with those experiences, and has made it through to the other side (whatever that side may be), or who has successfully completed an adoption, knows the truth of this statement. This does not make the journey from one side to the other any less difficult, or any easier to comprehend as one travels. Tending the tree of life is often excruciating work. A tree of life, however, is the experience of both Eden and the Heavenly Jerusalem, and according to Revelation, its leaves are "for the healing of the nations" (Revelation 22:2). However the journey of "hope deferred" ends, it is my deepest wish that worship and preaching can help lead to the kind of healing that ultimately comes from God, who tends the tree of life with us. I offer this book with the quote from Proverbs as a guiding metaphor for the work of preaching and worship and it is my hope to provide resources for those who plan and lead in public worship and preaching. As pastors, preachers, and planners/leaders of worship, we stand alongside those charged to our care, tending the tree of life with them in public worship in addition to the many other locations of our ministries.

TASKS OF PREACHING AND WORSHIP WITH REPRODUCTIVE LOSS AND ADOPTION IN VIEW

With my story foregrounding the place from which I write, the primary goal of this book is not to promote theological views that definitively resolve the heartache, questioning, or even joy that is a part of those who tend the tree of life. Rather, it is my desire to begin breaking up the silences and unhelpful practices that make people like me feel as if we are in the shadows of faith communities and to begin moving individuals, families, and communities of faith toward better understanding, healing, wholeness, and faithfulness. I hope to help ministers and congregants grow with one another in ways that open up preaching and worship as events where all can grow in understanding and move toward healing. As such, this is primarily a book for pastors who lead faith communities in preaching and worship. But it is also my hope that individuals and small groups might also be able to use this book for their own purposes of healing, discussion, or to help bring about awareness for their ministers or other members of their faith communities. I now move to a large-scale pastoral framework for preaching and worship with reproductive loss and adoption in view.

Healing and Wholeness in Preaching and Worship

Why "healing" and "wholeness"? If you were to spend any time around institutions of theological education now, you are likely to recognize these two terms as theological buzzwords. As such, I am wary that they might be received as vacuous, overused terms that communicate less about their meaning and more about the fact that they are the right terms to use.

I use the term "healing," however, in the way that homiletician Kathy Black uses it in regard to disabilities: "Disability is a part of everyday existence for millions of people and their loved ones in this world...When cure is not currently possible, healing can happen through the supportive, accepting community; through our own ability (undergirded by God's strength and the support of others) to make it through the hard times; and through the different, new possibilities that are open for us."[2] Clinically, reproductive loss does not fall under the category of disability, but there are some similarities in that the body has failed to meet expectations of "normal" functioning. Furthermore, Black makes an important distinction between "cure" and "healing." On the one hand, cure would be the elimination of disability, or for our purposes the elimination of the causes and results of reproductive loss. Healing, on the other hand, entails the process of "making it through the hard times" and realizing the "new possibilities" that are present for us when our original hopes and dreams of biological children have been fractured or ruptured adoption scenarios occur. Part of healing, as Black describes it, is a kind of triangle that consists of the coming together of (1) a supportive community that helps (2) individuals survive, cope, and thrive while also connecting them to (3) God and the resources of God.

Individuals who have experienced reproductive loss or who are currently grappling with reproductive difficulties are often in need of healing. In all likelihood, the hope and search for "cure" has left them with significant wounds. Like many of the biblical characters explored later, if they have encountered silence, avoidance, injurious sacred texts, and/or unresolved theological themes, then the need for healing is compounded.

Similarly, there will be a search for "wholeness." The English word here correlates to the Hebrew word *shalom*, which can also

---

2   Kathy Black, *A Healing Homiletic: Preaching and Disability* (Nashville, TN: Abingdon Press, 1996), 42.

mean peace, health, and/or completeness. As someone who experienced a palpable void, the absence of a biological child, an absence
of God, and the evacuation of hopes/plans/dreams/expectations, I
can attest that in a very real sense it can feel like there are missing
pieces to the self. In my experience, whether some of the pieces of
myself needed to be rearranged or some needed to be restored or
different pieces needed to fit into the voids or I needed to learn how
to cope and exist in a different state of being, I craved "wholeness."
Part of the work of preaching and worship as it relates to reproductive loss, I believe, can be the work of extending the possibilities of
healing and wholeness.

   Why do this publicly in the context of congregational worship? I recently read a quote from a leader in theological education
that said, "Real ministry happens not in the pulpit, but where the
people are and where they are hurting." This statement is problematic in a number of facets, but most notably for our purposes, it
expresses the erroneous assumption that preaching (and worship)
are incapable of addressing the contexts ("where the people are")
and pastoral needs ("where they are hurting") present among those
gathered for worship. The quote betrays a severe lack of confidence
in the power of preaching and worship to do significant ("real")
pastoral work.[3]

   For a moment, let's take the bait. This thought gives rise to
at least one significant question about the relationship among different ministerial practices. If people are hurting with these issues,
shouldn't healing take place in the confines of pastoral counseling,
group counseling, and one-on-one with psychologists and psycho-
therapists? Yes. Without a doubt, people should avail themselves of
the full range of therapies available to them in settings that make

---

3   Incidentally, this was a question that surfaced in a large way in the late
    1960's concerning the effectiveness and role of preaching, just prior to
    the original release of Fred Craddock's Fred B. Craddock, *As One without
    Authority*, Rev. ed. (St. Louis, MO: Chalice Press, 2001). Craddock's
    work, and that of his peers, in what is now known as "the New
    Homiletic," significantly changed the perception about the loss of power
    related to preaching. It is interesting that this question has surfaced again.

them comfortable and allow them to process thoughts and feelings in significant ways. There are tremendous possibilities for healing and wholeness within the range of those practices that fall under the rubric of "pastoral care." However, preaching and congregational worship possess a public dimension that holds possibilities for different avenues toward healing and wholeness. The church's preaching and congregational worship are two of its most public "faces," and the opportunity to engage in communication and communal liturgies intentionally structured toward meaning-making, healing, and developing a community of care should not be avoided simply because the topic is deeply personal and difficult. This is not even to begin breaking the surface of exploring how communities of faith believe preaching and worship manifest God's word, God's promises, the cross, and resurrection in the midst of the congregation.

Theological Naming and Local Theologies

One other preliminary defense of addressing reproductive loss and adoption within the public context of congregational preaching and worship: these two public, congregational practices provide an opportunity to engage in "theological naming" and "constructing local theologies." In terms of theological naming, the words of Christine Smith are especially powerful:

> Preaching is an act of public theological naming. It is an act of disclosing and articulating new truths about our present human existence. It is an act of bringing new reality into being, an act of creation. It is also an act of redeeming and transforming reality, an act of shattering illusions and cracking open limited perspectives. It is nothing less than the interpretation of our present world and an invitation to build a profoundly different new world.[4]

---

4   Christine M. Smith, *Preaching as Weeping, Confession, and Resistance: Radical Responses to Radical Evil*, 1st ed. (Louisville, KY: Westminster/ Knox Press, 1992), 2.

While Smith's specific goals are addressing injustice and evil, her statement applies to the dimensions of preaching and worship addressed here. Ron Allen likewise defines preaching as "theological interpretation."[5] Preaching and worship with reproductive loss and adoption in view can participate in the rebuilding of shattered realities and the imagination/construction of new possibilities in people's lives. Pastoral theologian Carrie Doehring calls this moving from largely un- or pre-reflective "embedded theology" to "deliberative theology" which seeks to make sense of experiences of loss, grief, and suffering.[6]

As a corollary to theological naming, preaching and worship attempts to construct local theologies. Nora Tubbs Tisdale adapts this phrase as a way of describing the work of preaching in local communities.[7] Rather than the preacher dispensing her theological wisdom from the resources of her study and disembodied theologians, the preacher works out of the resources of her location. Preaching is an act of constructing "local theology," crafted for a particular people at a particular time and place. To do this, the preacher engages in congregational exegesis/study (a form of localized anthropology) which identifies the symbols and narratives that reveal cultural and theological identity, providing interpretive frameworks through which the local pastor can deepen her understanding of the congregation's worldview, values, and ethos. The goal is engaging in contextual preaching, which takes the culture in which one preaches as seriously as one takes the proclamation of the message. The preacher stands as a kind of ethnographer within the congregation.

If this is one of the roles of the pastor, then preaching and worship with reproductive loss and adoption in view means that the preacher will do extra work to identify the symbols and narratives

5   Ronald J. Allen, *Interpreting the Gospel: An Introduction to Preaching* (St. Louis, Mo.: Chalice Press, 1998).

6   Carrie Doehring, *The Practice of Pastoral Care: A Postmodern Approach* (Louisville, Ky.: Westminster John Knox Press, 2006), 112ff.

7   Leonora Tubbs Tisdale, *Preaching as Local Theology and Folk Art*, Fortress Resources for Preaching (Minneapolis: Fortress Press, 1997).

within a particular locale that help provide interpretive frameworks through which congregants can process their questions and heal from their wounds. This means that preaching, liturgy, and theological formulae will vary from place to place and time to time. It also presents an opportunity for pastors to engage in fresh interpretations of what is going on *alongside* congregants (because local theology requires deep listening), rather than simply *for* congregants.

The Role of the Minister

Related to this, I want to advocate that preaching and worship with reproductive loss and adoption in view requires a particular way of envisioning the disposition/role of the pastor. Some will be familiar with Tom Long's work in his introductory preaching textbook that raises the importance of the image of the preacher. He seeks to add complexity to the images of "herald" and "storyteller" and proposes that the preacher envision herself as "witness." This image retains a large focus on the authority, agency, and knowledge of the pastor, even as he suggests that the pastor "rises from the pews" in solidarity with congregants.[8]

I believe a more appropriate image for how the pastor envisions the work of preaching and worship is in order for the specific pastoral situation under consideration. John McClure describes the role of the preacher as "host and guest."[9] Without digging too deeply into the philosophical and theological roots of McClure's image of the preacher, we can see that this image positions the preacher as one who "hosts" the processes of preaching (and planning worship) as well as plays the role of "guest" among different voices who extend the preaching conversation to territory that the pastor may or may not know. As such, the preacher is one who does not just

---

8   Thomas G. Long, *The Witness of Preaching*, 2nd ed. (Louisville, KY: Westminster John Knox Press, 2005). 3.

9   John S. McClure, "Preacher as Host and Guest," in Robert Stephen Reid, ed. *Slow of Speech and Unclean Lips: Contemporary Images of Preaching Identity* (Eugene, OR: Cascade Books, 2010), 119-43.

emerge from the study with words from on high (or even from the pew) to dispense wisdom to those who experience reproductive loss or the various stages of adoption. Instead, the pastor opens up the preaching process as a *listener*, as someone who is willing to allow the other guests to move into the position of host (even if only for a short while) to learn from their experiences and viewpoints. By allowing the pastor to listen to the stories and questions of worship participants (with permission, of course), those who have not experienced reproductive loss are able to access and listen to the community's deepest concerns. Working within the framework of this image, the preaching (and worship planning) process becomes one of mutuality, even as the pastor will ultimately construct and preach the sermon or often be the one who leads and plans worship.

Communities of Care and Pastoral Communication

Once a pastor makes the choice to break silences, avoid avoidance, and engage theological themes (which will be discussed later), opportunities for pastoral dimensions (with the goals of pursuing healing and wholeness) of preaching and worship are present. There are two models that set an appropriate agenda for engaging reproductive loss and adoption in preaching and worship. By this, I mean that there are some overarching goals in terms of the kind of preaching that will take place with reproductive loss and adoption in view. Other than pursuing healing and wholeness and engaging in a specific type of preaching disposition/role through theological naming, constructing local theology, and embodying the image of the host/guest, pastors have a responsibility to the dynamic of both congregations as a whole and to individuals/family units.

The first of these goals is to establish/form a community of care. Silence and avoidance leave people who are experiencing reproductive loss and striving for adoption as isolated, distant, and without a safe public space in which to reach toward healing and wholeness. In other words, the work of healing and wholeness for those who experience reproductive loss becomes relegated to the sphere of individuals' private lives. We do not do this with other kinds of losses experienced in congregations. Let me be clear here: preaching and public worship that address reproductive loss and adoption will not attempt to single anyone out or break the confidence of private pastoral conversations. But it will attempt to formulate preaching and worship that (1) acknowledges the reality of reproductive loss or losses in adoption *as loss* and (2) provides resources toward healing and wholeness for individuals, family systems, and congregations.

Lee Ramsey describes the formation of pastoral community as dependent upon three interrelated categories of pastoral work: (1) mutuality in ministry, (2) hospitality, and (3) care/compassion for the world.[10] Regarding mutuality in ministry, Ramsey believes that preaching (and the focus of his work is primarily on the practice of preaching) works to form the kind of community that works to connect people in relationships where they are responsible for the care of one another. He makes a point significant for our purposes: "Pastoral communities do not exist for the primary purpose of making individuals get over whatever ails them...Members of the Christian pastoral community edify the community as a whole.... We are shepherds of the common good of the community, each one contributing his or her pastoral gifts for the caring nature of the entire fellowship."[11] Preaching and worship will strategically seek to develop the kind of community that empowers people to minister to one another not just *in* but *beyond* instances of congregational preaching and worship.[12]

Pastoral communities also seek to embody the kind of hospitality that encourages people to fully bring all of who they are to all of who God is in the practices of Christian preaching and wor-

---

10 G. Lee Ramsey, *Care-Full Preaching: From Sermon to Caring Community* (St. Louis, MO: Chalice Press, 2000), 31-58.

11 Ibid., 48.

12 I will say more about what I mean by using the word "strategic" below, but I use this word intentionally here.

ship.[13] We have already expressed the importance of the preacher
taking up the image of preacher as "host/guest." This implies that
the pastor embodies the kind of hospitality that fosters a community of care for those seeking healing and wholeness. Ramsey says that
"hospitality is an act of Christian care on behalf of the outsider who
seeks prayer, shelter, food, strength, and human companionship.
The pastoral community offers hospitality to the stranger because
it is the nature of the community to do so. Having received the
hospitality of Christ, who is the host of Christian worship and
thanksgiving (Eucharist), the pastoral community incorporates
hospitality into itself and becomes the hospitable community for
others."[14]

A quick example may help make the point about hospitality.
When my wife and I were looking for a church to attend while I
was in graduate school, not active in pastoral ministry, and were
experiencing reproductive difficulties, we were often greeted before
worship officially started or during the passing of the peace (by
both clergy and laity) first by asking our names, then immediately
followed by the question, "Do you have children?" This sounds
innocent enough, until you have experienced reproductive loss
and are wrestling with your personhood before God. It felt as if
our personhood was being overlooked in an effort to garner more
children in the children's ministry. This question often screamed
out to me that a congregation saw us as fresh meat. I recognize that
intentions were innocent, but their innocence did not change how I
felt. Ramsey makes a similar distinction regarding Christian hospitality: "Hospitality…is not for the purpose of meeting institutional
goals—more members, a bigger budget, more people to support
our programs."[15] I consider greetings prior to the "official" start of
worship an integral part of congregational worship. But developing

---

13   Again, I echo Don Saliers' definition of Christian worship as the human
     pathos meeting Divine ethos, Don E. Saliers, *Worship as Theology:
     Foretaste of Glory Divine* (Nashville: Abingdon, 1994).
14   Ramsey, *Care-Full Preaching,* 50.
15   Ibid.

hospitality within a community of care means being aware that people enter into the context of worship with specific needs and wounds that a simple, unreflective greeting might exacerbate, and adjusting our practices accordingly.

Finally, Ramsey raises the dimension of care/compassion of the world as a goal for preaching. By adding the component "of the world," Ramsey suggests that preaching (and worship) possess the capacity to form a community that is both interested in and actively pursuing ways of healing the world beyond the doors of the local congregation (and the people within them). This dimension also recognizes that those inside the doors of the local congregation are an integral part of the world beyond those doors.

Reproductive difficulty/loss and adoption extend beyond the internalized emotional experiences of individuals to the impact of broader societal systems. For instance, what kinds of reproductive medicine and consultation does an individual's health insurance policy cover, if any at all? How can those without the means to pay for reproductive medicine resolve their desires for biological children in the midst of a cultural framework that so highly values (and exerts pressure to achieve) biological children? What are the financial, legal, and social barriers to adoption? Reproductive difficulty/loss and adoption occur within a complex societal framework of which we are all a part.

As Ramsey says, "Communal care rests on the theological conviction that world and church, individual and society, are united in God's Kingdom; all express the fullness of creation that God intends. To heal the world is to heal the individual in the world. To express care within the church is to contribute to the wider environment of care that extends to the end of the earth."[16] Preaching and worship that develops a community of care will seek to express the knowledge that reproductive difficulty does not happen simply within the confines of the individual's body and mind nor adoption within a nuclear family unit, but in complex systems to which we are all called to attend.

---

16 Ibid., 57.

The second goal consists of creating effective pastoral communication. J. Randall Nichols suggests two important components that might shape our understanding of what preaching and worship intend for individual and congregations. The first is that "preaching as pastoral communication" works toward "restoration."[17] Nichols intentionally phrases the term "preaching as pastoral communication," which is worthy of unpacking in a small way here. By using the term "communication," Nichols seeks to integrate the insights of studies in communication more than, as he says, "the traditional concept of 'homiletics' easily allows."[18] Here is where the term "strategic" becomes important. Preaching as pastoral communication conveys the importance of intentionally structured congregational rhetoric. Intentionally structured congregational rhetoric hopes to achieve small-scale and large-scale goals, both for individuals and for congregations as whole.[19] This does not make preaching a wooden or manipulative activity, but insists the pastor be conscientious about the goals and intended impact of preaching and worship. As it relates to reproductive loss and adoption, pastors will want to be strategic about the intended impact of the rhetoric of preaching and worship, carefully envisioning ways she hopes to create a community of care.

Preaching as pastoral communication, according to Nichols has as one of its goals, "restoration." I believe that this word is closely related to "healing," discussed above, but it introduces an element of time that is an important function of encountering reproductive difficulty and loss. According to Nichols, "restoration carries a dual commitment to past and future, old and new, here and elsewhere...The work of restoration is neither losing the past nor living in it but rather creating a present that reaches realistically out to both past and future. Restoration is neither harsh confron-

17 J. Randall Nichols, *The Restoring Word: Preaching as Pastoral Communication*, 1st ed. (San Francisco: Harper & Row, 1987).

18 Ibid., 12.

19 For a larger treatment of the strategic communication of preaching, see John S. McClure, *The Four Codes of Preaching: Rhetorical Strategies* (Louisville, KY: Westminster John Knox Press, 2003).

tation of the inadequacies of what and whom we deal with nor passive acceptance of them; it involves the creation of something new that both acknowledges its ancestry and embraces the growing yet to come."[20]

Several items are important to highlight here. First, by addressing reproductive loss in preaching and worship, we are not trying to encourage forgetting a painful past or present. Past and present are valued, even as painful experiences, but they do not keep those who suffer as hostages. Second, the work of restoration acknowledges that there is a future different from the past and present, and works toward shaping that future. Third, the shaping of that future requires agency and activity. Preaching and worship will help to reshape the sense of agency and control that those who suffer reproductive loss no longer possess. Finally, although Nichols' use of the word "ancestry" is certainly incidental, it conjures up a notion of family that is particularly important for our purposes. The work of restoration in relation to reproductive loss and adoption means that the past dreams of ancestry and future ones will likely be forged in new and/or different ways than we first imagined. As pastoral communicators, we will want to preach and plan worship in ways that work toward restoration, helping people tie together in new ways the past, present, and the future.

The second component from Nichols is closely related to Ramsey's idea of fostering a community of care. In describing the communal effects of "pastoral communication," Nichols states that "what will be created by a given sermon—or, more likely, by a longer term of preaching—is partly within the control of the preacher. By knowing something about the options we can begin to be more strategic and more intentional in planning our pastoral preaching. The basic idea here is that *messages create communities*, or as it is sometime said in communication jargon, publics."[21] Certainly this ties to the idea that pastors are in the work of constructing "local theologies" by learning from the symbols and narratives at work in

---

20 Nichols, *The Restoring Word*, 4.
21 Ibid., 103.

a community, but Nichols turns this around in the other direction, emphasizing the rhetorical force/effect of preaching as possessing an inherent ability to create a kind of public.

As such, we should not only be aware of this effect, but intentional about using it to achieve some kind of desired result. Nichols makes a case that the intentionality of pastoral communication in preaching (and similarly in worship) has both an ecclesiological outcome and a pastoral outcome. We will create one kind of public or another. That public will include some and exclude others. That public will work toward some pastoral goals at the exclusion of others. Not every sermon can be "all things to all people," but the strategic pastor will attend as much to sermon content as she will to "the kind of community that is structured…Our pastoral work and wisdom, in other words, rests at least as much on this field-structuring dynamic as it does on the cleverness or profundity of what we say (though, of course, the two are intertwined)."[22] The reason we are laboring here before getting to the more specific tasks of "what to say" is so that we can be intentional about determining the kind of congregational public we are creating. The sense of being part of a restoring/restored public can be as powerful as hearing affirming content in a sermon or moment in worship.

Preaching and worship with reproductive loss and adoption in view is as much communal as it is individual, as much congregational as it is societal and even global, as much about inhabiting/embodying a new image of the pastor as it is about developing a new way of talking about a difficult subject. To boldly incorporate reproductive loss and adoption into these pastoral tasks requires a strong sense of what it is that we are trying to accomplish within our faith communities. With these broader goals in mind, we now turn to how preaching and worship can faithfully address reproductive loss (chapters one and two) and adoption (chapters three and four). At the end of the book I provide an appendix with portions of sermons and worship items that I have used within my own congregational ministries.

---

22 Ibid., 105.

Chapter One:

Silence, Texts of Terror, and Images of God

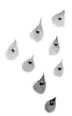

For those who preach or lead worship regularly, when was the last time a sermon or public prayer of yours addressed reproductive loss? When was the last time you preached even part of a sermon or prayed in a public worship service about the difficulties of conception, miscarriage, stillbirth, etc.? When was the last time you even thought about these experiences as they relate to worship or preaching? Perhaps you can sense the awkwardness you or your congregants might feel if these issues were to become part of public worship. These are difficult issues. And the ten to fifteen percent of couples who face infertility issues[23] and those who experience the one in five occurrences of miscarriage[24] will rarely, if ever, encounter preaching and worship that addresses these significant life issues. As we consider how preaching and worship function with reproductive loss in view, I begin by exploring three major issues: silence, texts of terror, and images of God. I will then outline some interpretive strategies for the work of preaching and worship.

The Problem of Silence

Silence is certainly the most obvious obstacle to preaching and worship as it relates to issues of reproductive loss, and it is perhaps also the most pernicious. Imagine walking into a house of worship weighed down with the emotional and spiritual questions these experiences carry with them and not being able to find a place to process those experiences. What is it like to never hear a word about such a significant part of one's identity and part of the human ex-

---

23 http://www.mayoclinic.com/health/infertility/DS00310, accessed February 18, 2013.

24 http://www.mayoclinic.com/health/pregnancy-loss-miscarriage/ DS01105, accessed February 18, 2013.

perience in such a formative time and space as Christian worship? If one of the purposes of preaching and worship is to explore what it means to be human in the light of who God is and what God has done, then silence about the issues that affect so many people leads to preaching and worship that does not completely fulfill its intentions.[25]

The issue, of course, is larger than just the purposes of preaching and worship. Silence on issues of infertility and fertility/pregnancy/reproductive loss leads to a sizable number of Christian worshippers being unable to locate themselves and their life experiences within the realm of Christian existence. At the risk of overstatement, this can feel like a loss of Christian personhood. Without any words to validate these experiences from the faith communities who inform us about who we are, particularly in relationship to God, it can feel as if this significant part of life is disconnected from the Christian community. And in fact, this silence can lead to isolation within otherwise powerful and formative connections in community.

Several questions surface for which there seem to be no answers offered: "What does scripture have to say about what I'm experiencing? What is God's role—if indeed God is present—in the midst of the suffering I'm experiencing? What role does the faith community play if there is no collective wisdom to be shared about what I'm facing? Is this part of my humanity not addressed by the faith community?"

These kinds of questions are not exclusive to issues of infertility and miscarriage. Feminist, African American, Womanist, Asian American, Latino/a, and a range of other types of biblical scholarship have been engaging the themes of silence and identity in regard to biblical interpretation, preaching, and worship for some time now. Naturally, this means that these interpreters have found a significant part of their existence denied in the realm of Christian worship and in public life. The dominant modes and perspectives of interpretation are largely Eurocentric, male, and heterosexual.

---

25 This definition is interpreted from Don E. Saliers, *Worship as Theology: Foretaste of Glory Divine* (Nashville: Abingdon, 1994), 22.

Other interpretive lenses have been silenced or marginalized. When only a portion of the human experience gains voice in preaching and worship, part of creation is denied its witness (or perceived lack thereof) to God in the world. If preaching and worship are to address the whole person and the widest varieties of human experience, then giving voice to reproductive loss joins the chorus of witnesses which seek to engage issues of silence in biblical interpretation.

TEXTS OF TERROR

Silence is not the only problem, but it functions as a root for others. Without the benevolent guidance of an interpretive community, a number of biblical texts can function as "texts of terror" for those who face infertility and fertility/pregnancy loss. Phyllis Trible's well-known category explores biblical texts that cause the reader injury from their telling. This is more complex than just being unable to find oneself and one's experiences within the sphere of Christian preaching and worship as a result of silence. Experiencing a biblical text as it is read, preached, sung, or otherwise used in worship as a text of terror is to feel it do damage to one's sense of personhood before God and others. As Trible says,

> To tell and hear tales of terror is to wrestle demons in the night, without a compassionate God to save us. In combat we wonder about the names of the demons. Our own names, however, we all too frightfully recognize. The fight itself is solitary and intense. We struggle mightily, only to be wounded. But yet we hold on, seeking a blessing: the healing of wounds and the restoration of health. If the blessing comes—and we dare not claim assurance—it does not come on our own terms. Indeed, as we leave the land of terror, we limp.[26]

---

26 Phyllis Trible, *Texts of Terror: Literary-Feminist Readings of Biblical Narratives*, Overtures to Biblical Theology (Philadelphia: Fortress Press, 1984), 4-5.

The Christian canon can indeed inflict a type of limp without certainty of healing or restoration. Even as we faithfully wrestle with these sacred texts, hoping that they will indeed at some point yield to us answers and comfort, they can leave us feeling wounded and alone. But which stories related to issues of reproductive loss might we include among these texts of terror?

Miracle Births

The biblical story is replete with miraculous births. The Genesis narratives, in particular, dramatize the difficulty of having children along with several births by divine intervention. Seven chapters describe how Abraham and Sarah conceive at an old age after nearly all hope is lost (Genesis 15-21). In fact, the salvation narrative of the people of Israel is built upon God's promise to Abraham and Sarah through the birth of Isaac. Isaac's wife Rebekah was "barren" as well, but she eventually conceived Jacob and Esau (Genesis 25). God plays a significant role in the child-bearing of Leah and Rachel, Jacob's wives. While Leah was rewarded with the birth of Reuben because she was loved less than Rachel, Rachel too was "barren." After much anguish and drama, Rachel finally conceives the great Hebrew leader Joseph (Genesis 29-30).

Outside the Genesis narratives in the Hebrew Bible, the Hebrew people on their way out of Egypt are promised that God "will take away sickness from among you, and none will miscarry or be barren in your land" (Exodus 23:26). Certainly this was not the case, was it? Later, in the period of the Judges, "there was a certain man of Zorah, of the tribe of the Danites, whose name was Manoah; and his wife was barren and had no children." Visited by an angel, this woman conceived and gave birth to Samson (Judges 13:2). Hannah's agonizing prayers, which are mistaken for drunken babbling by the priest Eli in the place of worship at Shiloh, are turned into the conception of the eventual prophet Samuel (1 Samuel 1-2). Samuel, of course, plays a key role in the events that shape the politics and faith of Israel. The Shunammite woman is blessed with a son simply for her hospitality toward the prophet Elisha (2 Kings 4:8-17). Psalm 113 lifts praise to God, who raises up the poor to sit with princes and who "gives the barren woman a home, making her the joyous mother of children" (Psalm 113:9).

In the New Testament, Elizabeth and Zechariah are depicted after Abraham and Sarah. Elizabeth is "barren" and both are "advanced in years." They are miraculously blessed with the boy who will become John the Baptist, the forerunner (Luke 1). And then, of course, the reader encounters the chief story of miraculous birth in all of scripture: a young Israelite girl named Mary is visited by an angel during her betrothal to a man name Joseph and told that she will give birth to a son. Though she has no sexual contact with Joseph, she does conceive. The son will be named Jesus and he will be the one to carry forward the promises of God's salvation. Yes, the person on whom the entirety of Christian preaching and worship is built is the product of God's miraculous, intervening work of conception according to the writers of the Gospels.

Childlessness and the Complication of "Barrenness"

Other texts are less miraculous and more severe. Leviticus assesses the man who lies with his uncle's wife and a man who takes his brother's wife as sinful. The consequence for both parties is that they will die childless (Leviticus 20:20-21). Michal, the daughter of Saul, criticizes King David for his unfettered dancing before the Ark brought to Jerusalem. As a result, "Michal the daughter of Saul had no child to the day of her death" (2 Samuel 6:23). Childlessness serves as her punishment. Though David's sin with Bathsheba yields a successful pregnancy, the child dies after only seven days of life (2 Samuel 12:15-18). The prophet Jeremiah says of King Jehoiachin, "Thus says the Lord: 'Write this man down as childless, a man who shall not succeed in his days'" (Jeremiah 22:30).

Mark 13, Matthew 24, and Luke 21 all capture Jesus' apocalyptic discourse, usually interpreted as referring to the destruction of Jerusalem in 70 CE. Jesus' warning is of danger for those who are already pregnant and have young children: "Woe to those who are pregnant and to those who are nursing infants in those days!" (Mark 13:17). The implication is that these women are in danger of suffering and losing their children in the days when this comes to pass. In fact, they "will have little hope of escape."[27] In Luke 20, a hypothetical situation of childlessness becomes an opportunity for some Sadducees to interrogate Jesus regarding the resurrection. Childlessness is not the focus of the conversation, revealing a callous, insensitive gathering of people. For those who question Jesus, the situation of childlessness serves as the springboard for inviting Jesus into a contentious conversation. Childlessness itself is of little consequence for them.

It is helpful to pause a moment and explore the term "barren" as a kind of implement for injury in these texts of terror. "Barren" or "barrenness" is used twenty-four times in the biblical text. Five of those uses are in the New Testament, while the remaining nineteen are found in the Hebrew Bible. In Hebrew, the word is *aqar/aqarah*, meaning "barren" or "without offspring." In Greek, the word is *steira*, with the additional meaning of "incapable of bearing children." These are also terms used to describe fields that do not yield crops.

Proverbs 31 compares four things that are never satisfied and are never able to say, "enough": the grave, the barren womb, land which never has enough water, and fire (Proverbs 30:15-16). Isaiah 54 personifies Israel as a barren woman, extolling her, "Sing, O barren one, who did not bear; break forth into singing and cry aloud, you who have not been in travail! ...For you will spread abroad to the right and to the left, and your descendants will possess the nations and will people the desolate cities" (Isaiah 54:1, 3; also quoted in Galatians 4:27). Similarly, Jesus emphasizes his point on the way to the cross, "For behold, the days are coming when they will say, 'Blessed are the barren, and the wombs that never bore, and the breasts that never gave suck!'" (Luke 23:29).

---

27 Morna Dorothy Hooker, *The Gospel According to St. Mark* (Peabody, Mass.: Hendrickson Publishers, 1993), 315.

Finally, though Peter is referring to the virtuous life, he says "if these things [virtues] are yours and abound, they keep you from being ineffective or barren in the knowledge of our Lord Jesus Christ" (2 Peter 1:8). Peter transposes this physical term to the key of the Christian life of virtue.

Miscarriage

Miscarriage also has a place in the Hebrew Bible. Exodus 21:22 describes the penalty for a fight that results in a woman miscarrying her child, "When people who are fighting injure a pregnant woman so that there is a miscarriage, and yet no further harm follows, the one responsible shall be fined what the woman's husband demands, paying as much as the judges determine." The law Moses brings down from Mount Sinai provides restitution for the injury caused, though the restitution concerns the value of the household and benefits the husband more than the psychological, emotional, and spiritual health of the wife who experiences the loss.

2 Kings provides an etiology for the water of the city of Jericho. The men of the city of Jericho approach Elisha and complain that while the land in pleasant, the water of the city is bad. Elisha throws salt into the spring of the water and says, "'Thus says the Lord, I have made this water wholesome; from now on neither death nor miscarriage shall come from it'" (2 Kings 2:21).

Quite the opposite occurs in Hosea 9. As the prophet Hosea prophesies against Israel, describing the ways that God will punish them for their sin,

> Like grapes in the wilderness,
>   I found Israel.
> Like the first fruit on the fig tree,
>   in its first season,
>   I saw your ancestors.
> But they came to Baal-peor,
>   and consecrated themselves to a thing of shame,
>   and became detestable like the thing they loved.

Ephraim's glory shall fly away like a bird—
    no birth, no pregnancy, no conception!
Even if they bring up children,
    I will bereave them until no one is left.
Woe to them indeed
    when I depart from them!
Once I saw Ephraim as a young palm planted in a lovely
meadow,
    but now Ephraim must lead out his children for slaughter.
Give them, O Lord—
    what will you give?
Give them a miscarrying womb
    and dry breasts.

Every evil of theirs began at Gilgal;
    there I came to hate them.
Because of the wickedness of their deeds
    I will drive them out of my house.
I will love them no more;
    all their officials are rebels.

Ephraim is stricken,
    their root is dried up,
    they shall bear no fruit.
Even though they give birth,
    I will kill the cherished offspring of their womb.
Because they have not listened to him,
    my God will reject them;
    they shall become wanderers among the nations.
                         (Hosea 9:10-17)

Miscarriage, pregnancy loss, reproductive loss, and loss of children are God's punishment for Israel's unfaithfulness. In this instance, unfaithfulness is cause for divine intervention in the reproductive processes of the entire nation of God's chosen people.

Making Sense of the Texts

What are we to make of this catalog of stories and themes from the Scriptures? These miraculous birth stories, when read, heard, or preached, may potentially slap the recipient in the face. To encounter the stories of miraculous conception and birth is to encounter narratives of divine intervention that do not seem possible or likely in contemporary settings. If others have been the recipient of God's favor—deserving or not—then why must I/we endure the unknown, the feeling of unfulfilled desire, of emptiness, of loss? Some of these characters (the women in particular) are lifted up as models of faithfulness and/or endurance through hardship and thus worthy to be imitated. Indeed they are, but should we expect similar results? If faithlessness is the root cause of God's punishment as in Hosea, am I so faithless as to incur a similar punishment from God? For those who experience difficulty in conceiving or to carry pregnancies to term, the question naturally arises: what is the measure of faith one has to muster to obtain God's blessing in this regard? What is deficient in me that I/we cannot achieve what so many others do so easily? Where is God's intervention in my situation?

Even for those who can intellectually and spiritually separate the issues of faith and fertility, questions of faith can sprout up as gnawing questions. Is the overarching message of the biblical text reliable in this instance? What deficiencies in my faith exist that might be setting up a kind of roadblock to a successful conception and pregnancy? Again, even when an individual knows/believes that there is no correlation between one's faith and the ability to bear children (yes, even for those of us with M.Div degrees, ordinations, and doctorates in theological disciplines), these kinds of questions can crop up as a possibility when no other answers are offered.

The word "barren" is particularly injurious, suggesting that a person's life and worth are bound to producing children. To be barren is to add nothing to the global landscape, to yield nothing of note or benefit for the world. This is a concept that speaks to a person's negative self-worth and can become an integral and unhealthy component of a person's self-image.

If silence results in an inability to process one's experience within a Christian framework, or at least the lack of adequate resources to do so, then the reading and preaching of these texts without attending to the real experiences that mirror them in the contemporary setting does injury to worshipers. Silence does nothing to resolve feelings of loss and spiritualizing texts does further injury. Both fail to resolve questions of faith that linger. Silence and uncritical interpretation inflict brokenness and pain rather than providing the resources necessary for personal healing and wholeness.

IMAGES OF GOD

Finally, and related to the texts of terror, we should also explore images of God that become problematic for people facing situations of reproductive difficulty and/or loss. There are images beyond the three that I will explore below, but these particular images cover a broad range of issues.

1. God as Father/Mother

The language of God as father is most often the image used of God in Christian prayer and is attested throughout Christian scripture. Many pray the Lord's Prayer in worship each week: "Our Father…" Those who sing the traditional version of the "Doxology" each week in worship also sing, "Praise Father, Son, and Holy Ghost. Amen!" Or similarly, the *Gloria Patri*, "Glory be to the Father…"

In seminaries around the country, students are exposed to "inclusive language" policies for language surrounding God. That is to say, if a student uses "father" language to describe God, she is also encouraged to use "mother" language to describe God or avoid gendered language altogether. This promotes a kind of sensitivity with regard to gendered understandings of God so that God does not take on exclusively male or female attributes. In a pastoral sense, this practice assists those who have faced abuse from fathers or mothers by preventing language that might lead to transference of abusive characteristics to God.

The care with which the gendered understandings of God have been handled is laudable. A problem remains, however, with understanding God, regardless of gender, as *procreative*. God seemingly has no difficulty in creating sons and daughters for God's self. God is infinitely fertile, with no obstacles to conceiving or bringing forth children.

It may be hard for someone who has not experienced reproductive difficulties or loss to understand, but for those who have, this can be a difficult image of God to process. Serene Jones offers a personal account that presents the situation more fully:

> It had been raining all morning, and the earth gave way softly as Wendy and I dug into it with spoons from her kitchen…Wendy had been bleeding for three days, and she looked ghostly; she had just miscarried an eight-week pregnancy (her fourth) and was grieving not only this present pain but also her dimming hope of ever having children. In her grandmother's handkerchief she had collected a few small remnants of her loss – a combination of bloody tissue and dashed dreams. We placed these in the earth and tried to think of something profound to say, but words would not come. Having spent years together in a women's group at our local church, we were accustomed to praying to God in the feminine. But today, lifting up prayers to "Mother God" seemed like a cruel joke, and we felt bereft as we struggled to find other theological images that might hold us in this moment.[28]

When it no longer makes sense to see God as motherly or fatherly, and those images have dominated our conceptualizations of God, how does one imagine God? Jones and her friend Wendy

---

28 Serene Jones, *Trauma and Grace: Theology in a Ruptured World* (Louisville, KY: Westminster John Knox Press, 2009), 127.

make it clear that for them, at least at that moment in time, the metaphor of God as mother had become what Lakoff and Johnson call a "dead metaphor."[29] Dead metaphors are metaphors in which entailments no longer hold true in context.

Sallie McFague's work in "metaphorical theology" makes it clear that our attempts to describe God are always done in metaphor.[30] But for those who experience reproductive loss, this kind of father/mother metaphorical God language can ring hollow or incoherent. Does that mean we abandon these metaphors? No, because they still suggest something about God's qualities of care, protection, etc. But we can be careful about the frequency with which we use the metaphor and the instances in which we use the metaphor, understanding that some may find certain metaphors to be wholly unhelpful.

2. God as "Giver of Life"

The Nicene Creed describes the Holy Spirit as "the Lord, the giver of life." Within a Trinitarian framework, how do those who experience reproductive loss imagine God as "giver of life"? If this is indeed true, why is it that God withholds the gift of life from some, while giving life generously to others? Does this only refer to spiritual life (and thus a kind of body-soul dualism)? This can be an especially difficult image for those who experience miscarriage, stillbirth, and pregnancy loss. Why would God give something so precious and so important then take it away? How could God be so cruel, so indiscriminate, so...unlike God?

As I relate in the Introduction, my own personal experience was that in the midst of our struggles to conceive, it seemed like our similarly-aged friends were having children with rabbit-like frequency and ease. This was problematic for how I imagined God as "giver of life." It felt like God was withholding that gift from

29 George Lakoff and Mark Johnson, *Metaphors We Live By* (Chicago: University of Chicago Press, 1980).

30 Sallie McFague, *Metaphorical Theology: Models of God in Religious Language* (Philadelphia: Fortress Press, 1982).

us. This was problematic in relation to the Sermon on the Mount passage (Matthew 7:9-11), "Or what man of you, if his son asks for bread, will give him a stone? Or if he asks for a fish, will give him a serpent? If you then, who are evil, know how to give good gifts to your children, how much more will your Father who is in heaven give good things to those who ask him!" Why was it that God seemed to be withholding one of the most basic, fundamental, and burning desires of my heart? Or why was it that God seemed to be indiscriminately picking and choosing who was able to receive the gift of life?

The question of this image of God comes down to making sense of God's involvement in our lives. In my case, I realized that I was wrestling with some more popular theological concepts from my childhood and the reality that God was not so involved in my life so as to be manipulating the processes of reproduction. There was no testing, no sense of God's timing, no exercising of God's will that provoked my frustration, despite what I continued to hear from some of my would-be counselors.[31] God's giving and God's taking away (Job 1:21) was unrelated to these biological processes. The image of God as giver of life will be one with which many who experience reproductive difficulty and/or loss will wrestle.

3. God as One Who Tasks Humanity to Populate the Earth

Most readers will be familiar with the image of God who tasks humanity to populate the earth. Genesis 1:28 describes the mandate as given to Adam from God: "Be fruitful and multiply, and fill the earth and subdue it." From an early age many are taught that part of the Judeo-Christian ethic is to fulfill this responsibility. For some, taking this word from God to Adam seriously as a contemporary command might seem a bit silly. But many go to great

---

31 I will say more about popular theology and the role of preaching/worship in the next chapter. For now, I simply want to raise how difficult this image is to understand and resolve.

lengths to fulfill that directive and feel pressure as active members of
faith communities to do so. Plenty of congregations actively focus
their energies on families with children. But where do people who
cannot conceive or who experience pregnancy loss fit in the scheme
of creation, the perception of God's desire for humanity, and within
family-with-children focused faith communities?

It is important to recognize the pervasiveness of this line of
thinking. The power of social expectation to have children is not
simply a religious construct, but is also deeply cultural and social.
Enmeshed in the hopes and desires to have biological children is
the religious narrative that comes from God's directive to Adam
and Eve. But there is much more. The white Christian settlers of
the new world in America had children not just to survive in a new
setting or create sustainable households, but to establish America
as a "city on a hill" through their children. Procreation was/is a
means of Christianizing the world and fulfilling one's part of God's
purposes for the world. In other words, having children – and
children who will be raised as Christian, specifically—is seen by
some as participating faithfully in God's mission. I do not want to
be too quick to dismiss that part of the American and Christian
narrative as a thread in the fabric of desire for children in people
of Christian faith.

Right or wrong, and if not in full, then in part, this can be an
active force motivating the desire for children. It can be difficult,
then, to see oneself as unable to fulfill this mandate. Again, the
relationship between individuals and God is thrown into question.
Why does God give this directive and not allow/equip all people to
fulfill it? "Doesn't God *want* me to have children?" This is another
problematic image with which to wrestle.

INTERPRETING TEXTS AND CONTEXTS

I want to suggest some interpretive principles for contending
with these difficult passages of scripture, themes that emerge from
these scripture texts, and the three dominant and problematic im-

ages that I describe above. As with many of the suggestions in this book, I do not believe that these will fully resolve the ambiguity or injury experienced by those who experience reproductive difficulty and/or loss. But I do believe that for pastors they provide some beginning steps toward awareness and resources for opening the biblical texts with the possibility of healing rather than injury.

1. Be aware that these are live issues and difficult for people among the congregation in which you serve.

Being involved in people's lives as a pastor necessarily involves being aware of people's challenges. In your congregation, the chances are high that there are people who are experiencing reproductive challenges, or have in the past. While these are pastoral situations that we most often do not talk about publicly, a starting point for the pastor is awareness of the likelihood of reproductive challenges in the congregation and being sensitive to these situations as interpretive opportunities.

These issues are not simply limited to the young adults in a congregation. Older congregants may still have painful memories and experiences of reproductive loss that will affect them in different ways as their peers experience the joys of becoming and being grandparents. A miscarriage that a couple remembers on a specific date each year, an inability to conceive, or other situations may continue to haunt them.

In one congregation I served, an older couple without children seemed to be emotionally moved each time something significant happened with children in the life of the congregation, but they seemed uneasy and uncomfortable expressing anything about it. The same kinds of reproductive technologies available now were not available then and adoption (though present among some of their peers) was not as socially acceptable then as it is now. Sadly, I believe that they had significant unresolved grief regarding not having children.

As you approach these passages and themes in the course of congregational life, know that congregants' experiences will touch these passages in a myriad of ways, and a fresh experience with one of these biblical texts may touch emotions that for a long time have gone unexplored, unrecognized, or unresolved. Awareness leads to finding the resources to come alongside congregants in the work of preaching and worship.

2. Break the silence.

Of course, I mean this in terms of a larger congregation setting, but I think it is also important for individuals and pastors to experiment with breaking silences. As you sit and read, try saying these phrases aloud: "Infertility," "Reproductive loss," "Pregnancy loss," "Miscarriage," "Barren." Go into your worship space and try reading them from the pulpit, the lectern, or from behind the communion table.

What did you experience when you said each phrase out loud? What power did each phrase have over you? What feelings did this exercise stir up in you? What associations occurred as you said each word/phrase? Write down any thoughts and feelings you had as you did this. Revisit your thoughts when you encounter these texts and themes in scripture.

If your experience was flat, then I imagine you will have some further work to do in exploring the emotional realm of reproductive loss. This is not necessarily a bad thing. There are some emotional places we cannot access if we have not experienced them ourselves. If this is the case, I suggest having some private, individual or small group conversations in safe spaces with those who have. Go through this exercise and allow the individuals' responses to help you understand more fully.

In the process of interpreting these passages and exploring these themes, saying these words aloud can begin a process of understanding and of empathy. Regular conversations with congregants or friends outside our spheres as pastors, who have experienced or are experiencing reproductive loss, can help us access space from which to more fully understand how biblical passages and themes can injure. Making an appointment to speak with a fertility doctor or OB/GYN in your area to get more information about what people go through to conceive or how doctors approach their patients from an emotional, psychological, and/or spiritual perspective might also be of benefit. Breaking silences requires being educated and informed so that we can helpfully interpret human need and sacred texts/themes.

For those of us who have experienced reproductive difficulty and/or loss and are in positions of pastoral authority, breaking up silences can be a powerful experience for our own healing and the role we play in others' healing processes.[32]

3. Do not avoid these passages just because they might be difficult.

This is obviously related to breaking silence, but there are some differences. Anyone who has been in a relationship of any type knows that avoidance, while it might well include silence, is fundamentally different from silence. Silence stems from ignorance or naiveté. Avoidance consists of intentionally distancing oneself from someone or something for any number of reasons. Congregants know when you are avoiding something, and they receive it as problem within the pastoral relationship. Avoiding the passages or themes surrounding reproductive difficulty or loss communicates our fear of exploring issues that are freighted with a great deal of emotional energy or that we feel awkward in speaking about these issues in a public setting.

Of course, interpreting these passages and themes, as well as the process of incorporating them into preaching and worship, will be difficult. But avoiding them just because they are awkward or

---

32 Though it will be important to distinguish the difference between what Randall Nichols calls "self-display" and "self-disclosure." J. Randall Nichols, *The Restoring Word: Preaching as Pastoral Communication*, 1st ed. (San Francisco: Harper & Row, 1987), 121-26.

difficult will leave some congregants feeling as if their humanity is outside the boundaries of preaching and worship. In the next chapter I will suggest strategies for preaching and worship that help us "avoid" avoidance.

4. Recognize the social location of the pastor and aim for "transgression"

Ron Allen expresses the importance of recognizing social location as a factor in biblical interpretation in contemporary settings. He says,

> awareness of the preacher's own social location and that of the congregation can be a resource that helps the preacher become aware of a wide range of dynamics in biblical texts, Christian doctrines and practices, and ethical behaviors, some of which have not been in the purview of male Eurocentric preachers and scholars in the modern mold. The power to image the world from the perspective of Others can help European males become more sensitive to such matters.[33]

When we raise the issue of biblical texts, theological themes, and biblical images of God in relation to reproductive difficulty and loss, we are saying that social location is an inseparable from any resulting interpretations. Similarly, men will likely interpret their experiences differently from women, middle class people will likely have different interpretations from those caught up in cycles of poverty or the very wealthy, and racial/ethnic differences will also play a part in how people interpret text.

Allen also describes the process of "transgression," or crossing borders and boundaries in biblical interpretation. By this, Allen means that interpreters can engage resources and perspectives outside their normal realm of expertise, social location, and personal bias. By engaging in transgression (respectfully and responsibly) in interpretive practices, "transgression may be an important Other

---

33 Ronald J. Allen, *Preaching and the Other: Studies of Postmodern Insights* (St. Louis, MO: Chalice Press, 2009), 79.

that can help the preacher and congregation recognize previously hidden interpretive possibilities."[34] For the preacher this might mean becoming conversant with a wider variety of disciplinary literature: medical and psychological literature, for example, can help expand understanding. It may mean conversations with people like doctors and nurses, people who have experienced or are experiencing reproductive difficulty and/or loss, people of different social locations, or seeking out literature (novels, short stories, poems) that describe these types of situations from particular perspectives.

If silence and/or avoidance have been the norm in congregational preaching and worship, then transgressing one's own borders respectfully is a way of beginning to overcome those pitfalls.

5. Avoid spiritualizing difficult biblical texts.

As we seek out interpretive strategies for the kinds of biblical passages explored above, we might be tempted to abstract our interpretations and "spiritualize" them in such a way that the issues of reproductive loss are obscured. For example, patristic interpretations of the Bible often proceeded under what is now known as the fourfold nature or four senses of Scripture. For those unfamiliar with this interpretive scheme, patristic interpreters examined biblical texts with four different lenses:

(1) The literal sense. This sense presents the least possibility of spiritualizing of the four senses of Scripture and will probably be most familiar to readers conversant with contemporary historical-critical methods. Interpretation in this sense attempts to understand what the biblical author(s) intended through attention to grammatical and historical features. In other places this is referred to as the "common sense" interpretation of Scripture. The danger here, while not spiritualizing in the strict sense, is drawing a straight line from "meant" in the ancient setting to "means" in the contemporary setting. In other words, because an interpretation was true to ancient Israel or the early church, so it is for contem-

---

34 Ibid., 108.

porary people of faith. This might leave little room for nuance regarding contemporary situations that ancient authors could not have imagined (which is certainly true in the case of modern reproductive technologies).

(2) The allegorical sense. Here we might begin to run into danger. The allegorical sense searches for the meanings behind biblical texts. The book of Galatians takes one of the texts we have deemed problematic and reads it allegorically. In relation to Abraham, Sarah, and Hagar, Paul says:

> For it is written that Abraham had two sons, one by a slave woman and the other by a free woman. One, the child of the slave, was born according to the flesh; the other, the child of the free woman, was born through the promise. Now this is an allegory: these women are two covenants. One woman, in fact, is Hagar, from Mount Sinai, bearing children for slavery. Now Hagar is Mount Sinai in Arabia and corresponds to the present Jerusalem, for she is in slavery with her children. But the other woman corresponds to the Jerusalem above; she is free, and she is our mother. (Galatians 4:22-26)

What is the danger of scripture interpreting scripture in this way? On the surface, it is not problematic. Paul uses allegory in the process of making a point about salvation. Imagine, however, sitting in a pew listening to the preacher interpret the story of Abraham and Sarah, wrestling with why God blessed them with children at an old age. Instead of addressing a pastoral point of contact, you hear an allegory about salvation with the characters serving as typologies in a schematic of salvation history. This is confusing and altogether unhelpful.

Now, as a side note we might ask, "Does *every* sermon that mentions miracle birth or barrenness or miscarriage or pregnancy have to speak to the situation of reproductive difficulty and/or loss?" Certainly not, but once the preacher begins to develop a safe space in which these issues are addressed honestly from time to time, then we are heading in the right direction.

(3) The tropological or moral sense. In this type of interpretation, the interpreter looks at the text strictly for moral instruction. Seeking moral instruction from the biblical text is not an evil thing, but we are seeking to "avoid avoidance." In looking at the passage from Hosea, if we were to interpret the passage strictly through the tropological sense, we would look at it simply from the standpoint that Hosea calls people to greater faithfulness and moral conduct to avoid God's punishment. People of faith should evade the example of Israel's conduct. While this is true, it does nothing to address the harsh words about the kinds of punishments God doles out as it concerns reproductive loss or the relationship between faithfulness and fertility.

(4) Finally, the anagogical sense. Here the interpreter looks toward God's future, specifically in relation to the end times and the journey to heaven. Here again, a strictly anagogical interpretation can lead to a form of avoidance. For instance, in interpreting the passage in Luke where Jesus engages with the Sadducees on the childless marriages and the resurrection, the anagogical sense directs our focus to the nature of heaven, the nature of the resurrection, and the correct approach in this life to the life after this one. An anagogical interpretation, however, side steps the reality of childlessness and extends the lack of pastoral care and attention already present in the passage itself. In this way, the anagogical sense becomes an opportunity for silence and avoidance.

A brief example of what I mean by "spiritualizing" the text (though not necessarily using the four senses): Ralph Klein's reflection on Genesis 15 for the lectionary website "Working Preacher" settles on this conclusion: "Genesis 15 recognizes that it is sometimes hard to believe when we are in bad situations. But God addresses our bad situations with promises that ring true to our needs, just as God doubled down on the promises to Abraham and Sarah. God lives up to his [sic] relationship with us by demonstrating that his news for us is indeed good, that he is willing to risk his very self so that we might believe."[35] Does this instance in the relationship between Abraham, Sarah, and God involve the problem of belief and the covenant? Certainly; we cannot avoid it. But the problem of childlessness, reproductive difficulty, and the obscurity of Sarah in this covenant-making episode cannot simply be explained away as the difficulty of belief. The pain of childlessness is pushed out of view in Klein's interpretive work, perhaps because it is such a difficult thing with which to wrestle in the context of a sermon or public worship.

I do not wish to eliminate these ancient methods of engaging biblical texts on the whole. They have proven useful interpretive devices for hundreds of years and have left much wisdom for the church. I am, however, suggesting that in situations of reproductive difficulty and loss they may not present the most helpful approach to interpreting the biblical texts that we have explored above. They can further exacerbate the confusing relationship between faith and fertility. Engaging in a fourfold nature interpretation might very well constitute a form of avoidance. I suggest dealing with the reality of these texts head-on (see below), rather than abstracting them to any of the four senses.

6. Attend to the social and cultural contexts of biblical texts

When avoiding spiritualization or abstraction of biblical texts and themes that address reproductive issues, it is also important to direct our interpretive energy in constructive ways. One of the ways to do this is to be honest about the biblical texts before us, attending to the social and cultural contexts out of which these texts have come. Again, Ron Allen helps frame this issue for us:

> The text is an Other. It had its own social location in antiquity and that location had its own integrity. In the ancient world a text or doctrine asked people to believe and do certain

---

35 "Commentary on Genesis 15:1-12, 17-18," http://www.workingpreacher. org/preaching.aspx?commentary_id=1599, accessed September 26, 2013.

things that were consistent with the historical moment of the text and with the cultural forms and mores of particular times and places. An interpretive statement of what a text in the biblical world asked a community to believe and do can be taken seriously when that statement could be *plausible from the standpoint of ancient culture, history, literary conventions, or social practices*...[T]he preacher respects the Otherness of the text and brings it into conversation with the congregation today. The preacher helps the congregation name what the text asked people in antiquity to believe and do and helps the community compare and contrast the social location and voice of the text with the social location and deepest theological convictions of the church today. The preacher can then compare and contrast the theological advice the biblical writer gave to the biblical community with the theological guidance needed by the contemporary congregation.[36]

By this advice, Allen helps us "avoid avoidance" of the biblical texts themselves. Instead, the preacher can dive headfirst into a respectful reading of biblical texts (notice that Allen includes doctrines as well, so we would include the biblical themes explored above) with critical interpretive tools that help assess the text as a document intended for a covenant community in the past while maintaining a dynamic (read: not static or straight-line meant/ means distinction) relationship through conversation with contemporary interpretive communities.

7. Attend to large theological themes

Finally, it is important to grapple with major theological themes that emerge out of experiences of reproductive difficulty and loss. We have already had some exposure to themes that emerge directly from the biblical texts. There are, however, more traditional theological themes that arise out of the experiences of reproductive loss and Christian faith. In interpreting biblical texts and themes, the pastor will also need to explore these themes. Though not ex-

36 Allen, *Preaching and the Other*, 82.

haustive, these themes are large enough to sustain quite a bit of reflection.

» Theodicy/Suffering

Theodicy and suffering are, of course, classic theological issues. In the course of a pastor's preaching and congregational worship, hopefully theodicy and human suffering will be addressed. The questions of theodicy and suffering are particularly acute through the experiences of reproductive loss. Why is it that God allows suffering and this kind of suffering, especially when others have relatively little to no difficulty conceiving or bringing children into the world?

The attentive preacher will attend to these difficult questions in ways that allows people to raise/voice their questions in safe spaces, help them explore a range of answers, and express care for them as they continue to make sense of their experiences through the lens of faith.

» Interpreting the Human Body

One of the major issues at stake when attending to reproductive loss is the actual, physical human body. Because we are created and creating physical bodies, the experiences of reproductive loss can produce a great many questions about what it means to be human. These questions are, undoubtedly, theological questions.

Kristine Culp suggests the term "vulnerability" as one which might be helpful as we think about the human body. She writes,

> The biblical notion that humans are creatures made of earth and breath likewise suggests vulnerability...Vulnerability encompasses not only the capacity to suffer harm and to be damaged, but also capacities implied to be healed and lifted. This robust notion of vulnerability can be read from the beginning to the end of the Bible in the stories of creatures who rise and fall, who make and break covenants, who are astounding

in their perversity and cruelty and also in their capacities to love and do justice.[37]

Those who experience reproductive loss will likely be able to identify with this theological term. The human body becomes a site of unpredictability, of the unknown, of openness to wound, death/the absence of life, and of suffering. The possibilities for transformation in and of the human body (Culp pairs vulnerability with the biblical term "glory" to talk about transformation) are uncertain. How do we make sense of Divine involvement in the human experience, or what Culp calls "life before God," when the human body experiences this capacity for being wounded and "glory" seems distant, if not impossible?

Serene Jones expresses four images of the self which she describes as "a drama of traumatic reproductive loss."[38] These four images express a great deal about how people experience the human body through reproductive loss.[39] (1) Control and responsibility/guilt. Despite cultural scripts of self-determination, reproductive loss brings about a "radical loss of agency" and "its counterpart: a sense of enormous guilt and responsibility for [the reproductive loss]."[40]

(2) A loss of a future. It does not take much imagination to see that along with the desire to have biological children, comes dreams about a growing life and one's relationship with it. Jones says,

> When a desired pregnancy fails—whether it is through a stillbirth or a failed in vitro fertilization—the woman experiences this known and yet unknown child not just as 'failing' but also as 'dying.' And with it dies a passionately imagined

---

37 Kristine A. Culp, *Vulnerability and Glory: A Theological Account*, 1st ed. (Louisville, KY: Westminster John Knox Press, 2010), 3.

38 Jones, *Trauma and Grace*, 134. I quote rather liberally from Jones here in an effort to avoid unfairly importing my male assumptions and interpretations too heavily onto a female-centered account.

39 Jones expresses that these are images that emerge from women's experience. I can say, however, that as a male I identify with some of these images as well.

40 Jones, *Trauma and Grace*, 135.

future, a future that is both the child's and the woman's. She thus grieves not only an immediate loss, but also the loss of an entire lifetime, a lifetime lived vividly in the drama of her hoping.[41]

While I admit having a different experience than that of a woman's in a failed IVF, this is not just a psychological loss, but a very physical one. Real cells and tissue that might have resulted in a life have been lost, along with all the hopes and dreams that might have been embodied with it.

(3) Jones identifies the third image as "loss of bodily integrity" or "the rupturing of self."[42] By this, Jones refers to a sense of the loss of a feeling of "borders" that separate the inside of the self from the outside. As what was inside the body (and for healthy pregnancies remains inside) moves to the outside, Jones hears women describe a sense of being unable to maintain pieces of themselves inside the borders of the body. Additionally, "for the woman who suffers infertility, this loss of bodily integrity is often the result of the constant invasion of her body by medical technologies that promise to extend her reproductive powers...This dissolution also happens to her each time she sees the unwanted blood of her cycle."[43]

Although men have different conceptions of inside and outside the body and the passing/exchange of vital bodily fluids in reproduction, this too is an image (albeit a markedly different one) that men may experience in the process of availing oneself of reproductive technologies.[44] Additionally, men may have a participatory role in the loss of bodily integrity experienced by female counterparts if they administer injections to their partners in preparation for reproductive procedures.

---

41 Ibid., 136.
42 Ibid., 137.
43 Ibid., 138.
44 For a dramatization of this male perception, see the character Toby Ziegler in *The West Wing*, Season 4, Episode 5, entitled "Debate Camp." He describes the process of giving a sperm sample for fertility treatments as "gruesome."

(4) Finally, the previous image is heightened as women experience their bodies as "spaces of death."[45] Women may experience their bodies not simply as places where life does not/cannot take place (a type of absence), but even more as a place where life is actively taken away. This is an experience of the human body that works against all religious and cultural scripts of motherhood.

As a person of faith, to experience the human body in the midst of reproductive difficulty and/or loss requires reflection on how one's body relates to God. I will say more about Culp and Jones' constructive theological proposals in the next chapter. For now, it is sufficient to suggest that these are at least some of the questions that are present when thinking about the human body as a theological topic in relation to reproductive loss.

» **The Silence of God**

Finally, the periods of waiting for good news, cycles of hope/despair, grief, and the practice of prayer that accompany reproductive loss and the pursuit of reproductive medicine bring to bear a question regarding the silence of God. If miracle births were brought on through Divine messengers and prophets in the biblical witness, then their absence suggests God's silence in individual contemporary experience.

In my own prayer life, while I waited between carefully timed ovulation cycles, induced ovulations via reproductive technologies, and then the eventual disappointments, I experienced a profound sense that God was silent and, at times, even absent. Although I was communicating and listening while waiting, I felt as if God, upon whom I was relying for guidance and comfort, was not returning the communication. This silence was compounded by the fact that I was finding few resources within the ecclesial setting for reflection on what I was going through.

What was I looking for in terms of a response from God? That is a difficult question to answer. It was certainly not an audible voice, but perhaps more of a presence – a feeling of peace to blanket

---

45 Jones, *Trauma and Grace*, 138.

over me in times of prayer when I felt most in turmoil or confused. I don't think this is too far from what others might long for in terms of communication with God. The silence can be unbearable and infuriating. My own theological conception of God's place in prayer was (and is) that God could "take it"—my anger, my confusion, my frustration—but the returning void did not even yield a still, small voice. And I was certain that I was listening.

Barbara Brown Taylor talks about the silence of God in this way: "What we crave in this wilderness are fresh words from the mouth of God—not yesterday's manna, nor tomorrow's, but just enough for today. Whatever happened to the talkative God of the Bible? What wouldn't we give for one comforting word in the garden in the cool of the evening, or a commandment so audible it made people cover their heads?"[46] Speaking into the seeming void of God's silence places a tremendous responsibility on those who preach and plan/lead public worship. The preacher should honestly address the silence and identify with the silences of God elsewhere in life.

CONCLUSION

It is my hope that this chapter has uncovered some of the issues at stake for those who are unfamiliar with reproductive loss, and that I have plotted a path for reflection on these issues. It has not been my intention to wrap them up in nice little bows with theological or pastoral resolution, and perhaps there is a heavy feeling at the end of this analysis. Pastors and local communities will need to work through these issues in the course of pastoral relationships and the practices of ministry. These feelings are complex, as is the week-to-week work of leading a faith community through preaching and worship each week. It is toward the practices of preaching and congregational worship that we now turn our attention. Through reflecting on the role of preaching and worship, I will take some of these themes and elaborate on the ways that they are turned

46   Barbara Brown Taylor, *When God Is Silent* (Cambridge, Mass.: Cowley Publications, 1998), 24.

toward more holistic/integrative responses (if not answers) to the problems outlined here.

Chapter Two:

The Roles of Preaching and Worship with Regard to Reproductive Loss

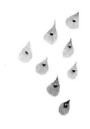

If, as we have seen, the major challenges for the church in regard to reproductive loss are silence, avoidance, injurious sacred texts, and unresolved theological themes, then it is incumbent upon pastors to help provide resources that can move those who experience reproductive loss toward healing and wholeness.

Tasks for Preaching and Worship

Although the distinction between what constitutes pastoral and prophetic ministerial practices can be somewhat artificial, in what follows I separate them for simplicity's sake. In describing pastoral and prophetic tasks of preaching and worship, I will use the word "help," perhaps to a fault. I believe that pastors' work in preaching and worship is part of a broader context of the "helping professions." That is to say, while pastors can open up conversations, introduce theological concepts/vocabularies, stir the emotions, and create a "communicative public," we cannot complete the work of healing for people, as much as we may want to, any more than we can make people engage in the work of social justice by their personal choices in everyday life. Preaching and worship provide resources, give aid, and create spaces for the work of healing.

Pastoral Tasks

1. Reaffirm personhood

One of the most fundamental tasks of preaching and worship with reproductive loss in view is to reaffirm the personhood of those who have experienced reproductive loss. When the human body, created in the image of God, has failed to do what it is biologically designed to do, there can be a sense of betrayal and that a piece of what it means to be human (again, created in the image of God) is missing or marred.

Again, Kristine Culp's idea of "vulnerability" is instructive. Part of our humanity lies in its imperfections. Our bodies break down, they are susceptible to inabilities and weaknesses. These are not defects in our personhood, though they may feel that way. Think back also to the "images of the self," as described by Serene Jones in the previous chapter. While not denying the reality of these self-images or the feelings that accompany them, we will want to offer affirmations that these self-images need not be permanent and that positive self-images of personhood are available through "life before God."

For instance, Culp begins her exploration of vulnerability and glory with the image from the Apostle Paul of humans as clay jars (2 Corinthians 4:7). She reflects, "Paul's deceptively simple metaphor of clay jars brings us close to the heart of the matter. It conveys a range of threats by associating malleable and breakable vessels with the dust of creation and of death. It signals, too, a range of possibilities: of creation pronounced 'good,' of everyday vessels suited for holy use, and of divine *pneuma* moving through and manifest in human life."[47]

The careful pastor will find a way to acknowledge in preaching and worship that our personhood before God does not depend on our physical abilities or our ability to bear children biologically. For those who, as Jones describes, feel that their bodies are bearers of

---

47 Kristine A. Culp, *Vulnerability and Glory: A Theological Account*, 1st ed. (Louisville, KY: Westminster John Knox Press, 2010), 17.

death, it is crucial to affirm that women and men are no less persons before God because they are not able to achieve or maintain a pregnancy. And just because we do not receive divine or miraculous intervention, this does not mean that God recognizes us any less. How our bodies function in the future may not be as we imagined them in the past, but there are different possibilities for the future that are most certainly inhabited by God.

2. Express care/concern while not offering easy answers

The idea of pastoral ministry as a "ministry of presence" is a well-worn path. It is important that pastors recognize that neither pastoral presence or preaching and worship alone will remove the pain and struggle of reproductive loss, nor will the answers offered up by pastorally-focused theological formulations remove difficult questions. The combination of these, however, can create a nexus in which care and concern of the pastoral community leads to healing and wholeness.

How do we do this in preaching and worship? At the risk of belaboring the point, it is crucial to break silences and avoid avoidance. Preach on the difficult texts and theological themes that relate to reproductive loss. At various points throughout the year, pray for fertility clinics, doctors, nurses, and patients. Pray for those who desire to have children but for some reason are unable to do so. While doing these things, refuse to offer up easy theological answers that deny the time and space in which people can process their thoughts and feelings. Deny the urge to resolve definitively the challenges people are facing. These difficulties are messy, and easy theological answers fail to express the care and concern required of long-term pastoral needs. We will explore some of those easy answers below.

When I began to preach sermons that at least in part addressed these topics, and incorporated these themes in worship, people seemed to experience more freedom in opening up to me as the pastor regarding these issues. The context of congregational worship became a place where healing could occur, or at the very least, a context in which people received the care and support of the faith community, without simple resolution. People are much more capable of living into the ambiguity and unknown of their lives when they know that they will be doing so in a place where they are loved and where their challenges are held in care by the pastoral community.

3. Help negotiate (not resolve) cycles of hope/despair

We briefly discussed in the previous chapter the presence of cycles of hope and despair. When reproductive loss is a part of one's life, the hope of procreation through sexual intercourse or reproductive technologies comes in regular, predictable intervals. Those trying to achieve pregnancy know well the personal schedules by which the processes of conception should take place as well as when menstruation (the obvious sign that pregnancy has not occurred) is likely coming. The periods of waiting are hope-filled, anticipating that pregnancy will be achieved (and that menstruation will not occur). They are counteracted by the moments when (and if) pre-menstrual symptoms arrive and, ultimately, when menstruation occurs. This brings with it moments of despair that once again the biological processes of reproduction have failed. When this happens repeatedly, cycles of hope and despair occur. For those who experience miscarriage, stillbirth, or other types of pregnancy loss (and especially repeated instances), the cycle of hope is prolonged as a result of an achieved pregnancy.

For those who have not experienced these cycles of hope/despair, consider for a moment the impact this has on an individual or couple. Doctors recommend attempting to achieve pregnancy through sexual intercourse for a year before pursuing any reproductive medicine. For those who experience reproductive difficulty and follow this instruction, this means that there might well be twelve cycles of hope and despair *before* seeking the help of reproductive medicine. The confidence placed in reproductive medicine "ups the ante" for cycles of hope/despair. The investment of time, money, bodies, and emotions beginning at testing/diagnosis and leading into procedures designed to increase the chances for achieving pregnancy heightens the sense of hope. Failed procedures likewise result in pronounced feelings of disappointment and despair.

The emotional, psychological, and spiritual toll that this can take on individuals/couples should not be underestimated. And the difficulty of pastoral work in the midst of these situations should not be underestimated either. In a congregation there may be people at many different points in the cycle. If there is a celebrated and physically noticeable pregnancy or birth while others are experiencing reproductive difficulty, then that may affect people's place within the cycle—even to the point of alternating between hope and despair from moment to moment. The cycles are not predictable or rigid.

The pastoral question for preaching and worship is "How do we help people negotiate cycles of hope/despair?" The image of the pastor as "host/guest" is important in this instance. Here the pastor has the opportunity to make preaching and worship an opportunity to allow the congregation to be a "guest" at other people's experiences of the cycles of hope/despair. This is not to say that we will put people's feelings and experiences on voyeuristic display, but moments of preaching and worship will acknowledge the reality of cycles of hope/despair and hold those moments before the pastoral community and before God. Access to these experiences, even when they are partial, provides an opportunity to develop a communicative public that recognizes what people are going through.

A question within a sermon as simple as "What is it like to be hopeful about something important, only to experience despair right on the heels of that hope?" might be effective for opening up this space. Similarly, a story (that does not have to center on reproductive loss) that helps people "overhear" the experience of cycles of hope/despair might prepare a safe space in which people can explore their own feelings.[48] For worship, a simple phrase within a

---

48 Fred Craddock is responsible for the term "overhearing the gospel." See Fred B. Craddock, *Overhearing the Gospel*, Rev. and expanded. ed. (St. Louis, MO: Chalice Press, 2002). While we do not want to equate human experiences or set up a false sense of "common human

pastoral prayer might open that space. For example, "God of hope, we pray for and with those who hope for the possibility of life… God who stands with us in our despair, we pray for and with those whose hope has been fractured…."

4. Help navigate grief/loss

Grief and loss are related to hope/despair. Grief and loss may accompany cycles of hope/despair. The inability to conceive, failed reproductive interventions (IUI, FaST, IVF, and others), and miscarriage all carry with them a profound sense of loss. Carrie Doehring describes six general types of loss: material, relational, intrapsychic, functional, role, and systemic.[49] Briefly, material loss would be the real physical loss, such as those associated with a woman's experience of a miscarriage. Relational loss would involve the loss of relationship, which might be at the very least a possibility for couples experiencing reproductive difficulty. Intrapsychic loss would include the loss of "whatever images that were formed of the child-to-be."[50] Functional loss would be the realization that one will not be able to have children biologically. Role loss might involve the end of relationships with trusted doctors and nurses. Finally, systemic loss would be the change in functioning of a family system or community because of how members of the system relate to one another or depend on one another. These losses are multidimensional. As with other types of loss that humans experience, reproductive losses are accompanied by grief and processes of grieving.

---

experience," (a widespread critique of the so-called New Homiletic) or using one experience to speak authoritatively for the experiences of all people, a facet of preaching and worship is offering up experiences, stories, and images with which people will be able to have multiple points of contact and/or identification. "Overhearing" is important because it may provide imaginative access both for those who have and those who have not experienced reproductive loss.

49   Carrie Doehring, *The Practice of Pastoral Care: A Postmodern Approach* (Louisville, KY: Westminster John Knox Press, 2006), 74-77.

50   Ibid., 75.

These losses and the grief that accompany them are all real—and we should not doubt that—though they are qualitatively different. The feeling of loss that accompanied our failed reproductive interventions resulted in a grief that, at times, blanketed our household. I do not want to equivocate that loss, however, with the loss of miscarriage or stillbirth. Nor do I want to compare these kinds of losses as measurably different. None are any more or less severe; they are simply different. In the interest of honesty, when my wife and I hear of someone experiencing a miscarriage or pregnancy loss, I experience our loss all over again, wondering what it might have been like to have been able to conceive and experience a pregnancy. I have a tough time imagining what it would be like to experience a miscarriage or stillbirth (from a male *or* female perspective).

The loss of hopes, dreams, and physical life are tremendous weights for people. Grief and loss are part of the human experience and we will all process them differently. The task of preaching and worship from the perspective of grief/loss is to help people navigate these places with the resources of faith. How does the pastor do this? Nichols suggests that the pastor creates a "holding environment" (which we also extend to congregational worship). He says,

> Both as a therapist and as a preacher…I hold the precious things my people bring—their histories, fantasies, hopes, relationships, worries, symptoms, all the rest. In the process, of course, I hold *them*, because that is the nature of a transitional object or experience: it carries part of the person himself or herself with it; that is how it does its work. I come more and more to realize that my skillfulness as a therapist does not depend so much on the experiences of my interpretations or the insightfulness of my observations as it does on my reliability as a "holder." The same is true when I preach. Even though here I am doing all the talking, I remind myself that, in effect, I am holding people through their concerns and issues, most

of which are unknown to me but which I inevitably touch with what I say.[51]

Here the pastor will feel the full weight of ordination (perhaps more as "host" than "guest" in these moments), but also the importance of being strategic in "preaching as pastoral communication." Preaching and worship at its best creates a public that allows congregants the permission to be fully present with their grief and loss. Congregational worship should not be a context in which people have to run from or hide the grief and loss they experience, nor will they have to rush through their grief to contentment or joy.

This can be accomplished in the process of the pastor building *ethos* with the congregation. Building *ethos* is a long-term project, but the pastor will project a type of pastoral presence over the course of a ministry. In the context of preaching and worship, the pastor will seek to develop an *ethos* that projects a message (verbally and non-verbally) that congregational worship is the kind of "holding environment" Nichols describes and that the pastor is trustworthy and caring enough to establish this environment.

5. Help identify God's presence and gift(s)

Finally, in the pastoral community it is of critical importance to locate God's presence and gifts in the midst of suffering and God's silence. Here the pastor is building a theological worldview (or local theology) for and with the congregation.[52] Through preaching and worship, the pastor will seek to help formulate, in the form of a theological narrative, answers to these questions: What is the role of God, if any, and where is God located in these situations? What specific acts/events/characters thwart a sense of the presence of God and reception of God's gift(s)? What is to be achieved (the goal) by

51   J. Randall Nichols, *The Restoring Word: Preaching as Pastoral Communication*, 1st ed. (San Francisco: Harper & Row, 1987), 82.

52   For more on building theological worldview as a task of strategic preaching, see John S. McClure, *The Four Codes of Preaching: Rhetorical Strategies* (Louisville, KY: Westminster John Knox Press, 2003). See especially the chapters entitled "The Semantic Code" and "The Theosymbolic Code."

the relationship of humans and God amid this kind of suffering? What shape do God's gifts take in these situations?[53]

As we have said previously, answering these questions will occur over long periods of preaching and worship in a community of care. Developing a consistent and solid narrative/theological worldview is a function of time through a pastoral ministry. On the other hand, however, the pastor will try to communicate answers to these questions in overt, specific ways in sermons and acts of congregational worship.

For instance, on the issue of suffering, the pastor can make clear that suffering does not mean that we are abandoned by God. God's presence in the midst of suffering does not protect us *from* suffering, nor does suffering indicate God's absence. Instead, God sustains us through our suffering, walking with us, tending the tree of life with us. These kinds of statements can be made in specific, unambiguous ways in preaching and congregational worship.[54]

Additionally, it is important to answer questions about the nature of God's gifts in the present and future. For instance: What do God's gifts look like when we must reorient our hopes and desires, especially if that reorientation includes coming to terms with the loss of the possibility of a successful biological pregnancy? What does/should the present as well as the future look like in terms of God's blessings in the face of reproductive loss, and what is God's role in bringing that about?

---

53 At first, I believed the correct term to use here was "grace," but this term was too laden in the language of soteriology as the correlating term to sin. I believe that "mercy" also participates in the language of soteriology. It is important to avoid the idea that reproductive loss is a function of soteriology. Instead, I will use the term "gift," indicating that God's presence with us always comes as gift. We might also use the term "blessings."

54 Again, see John McClure's description of the "semantic code" of preaching.

PROPHETIC TASKS

I now turn our attention to a sense of the prophetic. Simply, I define these prophetic tasks as a kind of theologically reflective "talking back" to dominant, often uncritically received cultural (and religious) scripts that send us messages about what we are to say, think, do, or be. The pastor can engage in the following kinds of prophetic tasks.

1. Help make sense of the use of reproductive technologies

This presents one of the most difficult challenges of all the tasks I describe for preaching and worship. There is no easy or non-jarring way to address reproductive technologies within the context of preaching and worship. Anyone who has entered a doctor's office or searched the internet and books for information on reproductive technologies will have had the experience of being introduced to an entirely new and overwhelming vocabulary. Statistics about success rates are alluring, even when doctors and nurses communicate clearly that success rates always indicate failure. There is a cultural script about the promise of scientific progress and medical intervention that gives us confidence in the possible use of reproductive medicine.

I want to name a few interrelated issues that coincide with decisions about taking advantage of reproductive medicine before I proceed to talk about the difficulty of addressing this within the confines of preaching and worship. The first issue is that of overcoming shame and/or anxiety when an individual makes an appointment for consultation with a fertility doctor. Men are usually suggested to be the first to visit a fertility doctor, which entails that men will have to admit some degree of failure. This is an affront to cultural scripts of masculinity, machismo, and/or male vitality, which prides itself on the capability of a man to successfully impregnate a woman and possessing (crudely, but culturally put) "strong swimmers." Men will have to negotiate giving sperm samples for examination and waiting for results about sperm count, morphology, and motility. Whether it is "right" or "wrong," results can be deflating to the male ego. Likewise, women will also have to admit the possibility that their bodies are not cooperating with dominant religious and cultural narratives about womanhood and motherhood. The initial appointment is an admission that something may be askew and that a woman might not be able to live into those narratives. A great deal of shame and/or anxiety can accompany this first step in availing oneself of reproductive medicine.

Second, there will be strong considerations of the cost(s) associated with reproductive medicine. There are wide variances as to what may or may not be covered under health insurance policies and the costs associated with reproductive medicine. For instance, under my graduate student insurance policy and my wife's insurance provided by her job as a public schoolteacher (which I would later join), both covered consultations and tests associated with diagnosing infertility, but nothing beyond this. As a result, after we went through testing and diagnosis (and there was some haggling with the insurance company about what this meant and what they would cover), we had to cover every penny of reproductive intervention without the assistance of insurance.

As a result, I personally had a difficult time wrestling with what was the wisest (and I use the term "wise" in the sense of faith, not simply in regard to a budget) use of our hard-earned money. At what point would spending money on procedures be too much or cross a line that was not clearly drawn? How did I express this as a husband who was also deeply sensitive to my wife's desire to achieve a pregnancy? What role did my faith play in the use of money for these purposes, particularly when that money could be going to do so many other things in the world? Why did it feel like we were trying to purchase a pregnancy?[55]

Related to this issue is the subject of class. Undoubtedly, reproductive medicine is limited to certain classes of people. Those

---

55 This becomes a complicated question for various kinds of insurance coverage, or lack thereof. While our insurance covered diagnosis and testing but no treatments, the feelings may have been different if insurance had covered the treatments as well.

without any health coverage will likely be unable to use reproductive technologies at all. The sophistication of reproductive procedures available will be dependent upon the availability of disposable income (often in significant amounts). I was deeply aware that class (and how class is intertwined with other social structures such as race) dictated what was available to me in terms of possibilities. My wife and I would not have been able to go through with our final and most sophisticated procedure, IVF, without having received some unexpected financial assistance. How we speak about reproductive technologies in preaching and worship will be connected to class.

A final issue is the medical manipulation of the human body. While I am not a Luddite regarding technology, manipulation of the reproductive processes of the body came with a wholly different set of implications than whether I should buy a smartphone with an Android or Apple operating system or even whether I should take an aspirin for a headache.

Admittedly, the medical interventions were not focused toward my body, but rather my wife's body. When faced with pills and injections (which I administered) that were designed to supplement hormone levels, time ovulation cycles, and when considering intrusive diagnostics and the engineering of embryos, I was faced with a dilemma. Was all this *ethical* within the range of my/our faith? When does life begin? To what extent did we need to share the same ethical vision/values as a couple when we made decisions on our use of reproductive medicine? Was tampering with the natural order of things somehow dangerous in terms of faith? An additional concern involved going through this as a couple. My answers to these questions might be different than what my wife felt were her own ethical limits. I had thought these things through *in theory* and had come to decisions that I thought were conclusive, but those decisions proved to be provisional as they slowly became real in the process of deciding together: "What will we do?" and "What are our limits?"

These interrelated issues, I hope, show just how complex attending to the issues of reproductive medicine in the context of congregational preaching and worship might be. Where does one begin to speak either as "host" or "guest"? How does the pastor pray and cultivate a community of care in relation to these deeply personal decisions?

There are two connected topics for preaching and worship that I think are most applicable here: wisdom and discernment. Congregational worship should be intentional about creating atmospheres where discernment and the pursuit of wisdom are cultivated. Rare are the occasions where the pastor will be able to directly address the ethics of reproductive medicine in the context of congregational worship and do it well. On the other hand, cultivating wisdom and practices of discernment can be done rather simply. If a pastor preaches in series, perhaps four weeks out of the year for congregational worship might focus on cultivating wisdom and developing discernment in a complex world. The focus of that search for wisdom and discernment could include several topics, not just reproductive medicine. It might trace biblical characters who sought to act wisely: Solomon, Ruth, Peter, Mary/Martha, etc. It might address someone like Hannah with an imaginative practice: "What if Hannah had lived today? Would she and Elkanah go to a fertility clinic? How far would they go to have a biological child?" Worship practices could include opportunities for worshippers to spend significant time in prayer, offering up the difficult issues of their lives to God and possibly even to the worshipping community, depending on the size and intimacy level of the congregation. Imagine the power of an individual or couple feeling safe enough to ask for wisdom and pursuing discernment on this topic in congregational worship.

2. Offer an alternative to the valorization of family

In congregations and American culture at large, we tend to valorize the nuclear family. The question we received at many congregations where we visited, "Do you have children?" and the order in which it was often asked, betrays the high value that congregations place on families with children. Let me be clear: I do not mean to say that congregations should *not* value the nuclear family. Christian tradition is clear that the church is responsible for nurturing the faith of all people. In light of my critique here, churches should not abandon their children's programming or cease to offer a Vacation Bible School in the summer.

The problem, however, is when "(nuclear) family" is valued or valorized so highly over different formations of "household." As pastors we will want congregational worship *and* the pastoral community formed by congregational worship to value all shapes and sizes of households, not just families with children. Some in the congregation will experience reproductive loss and never have children, biological or otherwise. This need not cause anxiety among congregants who cannot make sense of or accept this because of dominant cultural narratives about how families should look. Individuals should never be made to feel as if they are marginal or that they don't fit because they do not have children.

We can carefully shape our preaching and worship to create a community of care, rather than isolating and marginalizing those without children. Here the dominant image slides back to "host," indicating that we are trying to extend hospitality in an otherwise inhospitable cultural (and possibly ecclesial) setting. The pastor can start by illuminating images and stories of types of households and different formations of family that do not center on the nuclear family. This is also important outside the realm of reproductive loss, in an age where the construction of households and families occur in such a variety of ways. To center our images of family in preaching and worship on the traditional nuclear family is to miss LGBTQ families, families of the so-called "sandwich generation," and more.

Related to this, the pastor should carefully analyze the illustrations, stories, and images that are present in her sermons. Take a group of ten to twenty sermons that have been preached over the last year and scan them for what they say about families. Do they celebrate the nuclear family to the exclusion of other formations of family? How might I preach positive images of the variety of ways that congregants form families? Every day in newspapers, television, and the Internet, we get a glimpse of positive stories from the variety of ways that people form family in the contemporary setting. Pastors would do well to be attentive to these stories and store them away for future use.

Pastors should also celebrate the roles of aunts and uncles (biological and otherwise) and those who serve in close, positive roles for children. Before I became a parent, I became an uncle to my older brother and sister-in-law's son. I relished this role (even more through the period in which we were facing reproductive loss), even though I lived a significant distance from my nephew. I know several individuals who serve as "aunts" and "uncles" as close family friends who play special roles in the lives of children to whom they are not biologically related. Pastors would do well to lift these people up in preaching and prayers as those who serve invaluable roles by contributing to the various formations of family.

3. Counter uncritical and hurtful popular theological responses

Finally, it is of dire importance to counter the uncritical and hurtful popular theological responses to reproductive loss that dominate the religious cultural landscape. I often refer to these kind of responses as "pop theology." The words "uncritical" and "hurtful" are important descriptors of pop theology. I use the word "uncritical" because it is often apparent that people have not completely thought through their theological responses to this kind of suffering, especially the implications of what they are saying. Instead, they seem to offer overly simplistic answers that they believe (1) solve problematic questions and (2) provide some sense of pastoral care. In my experience, often these answers were offered without having asked for theological answers. I also describe these responses as "hurtful" because the answers themselves inflict injury to the individual. They cause injury to relationships as well. When I open myself to someone else with the details of reproductive loss and they respond with (unsolicited!) pop theology, I trust them less with my inmost thoughts, the details of my loss, and my questions. I should also add that these are all responses that I have heard and continue to hear in relation to reproductive loss.

What is pop theology in relationship to reproductive loss? Pop theology consists of answers given to those who experience reproductive loss that depend on variations of "sovereignty myths." Sovereignty myths integrate a very strong sense of God's agency and activity in every dimension of individual's lives. This manifests in at least three ways. The first is an umbrella category that responds to reproductive loss with the concept of "God's will." When people respond to individuals experiencing reproductive loss with the idea that this is "God's will," this entails that God is actively manipulating the normal biological reproductive processes in individuals and not only that, but actively denying people children. The image I use to describe the God who exercises God's will and sovereignty so far as to cover individuals' reproductive process is one of God as "puppet master" who manipulates human beings as a puppeteer would a marionette, pulling strings attached to the body to make it accomplish what God desires for it. This image of God is unappealing and imagines an intrusive, if not cruel God who stands in the way of successful pregnancy.

Why would God do this? This leads to the second and third of the sovereignty myths. God intervenes in the reproductive process because all things happen on "God's time." Under the umbrella of God's will, "God's timing" suggests that God has a secret, hidden schedule for human reproduction and that as humans our ability to understand that schedule is nearly impossible. For someone who has just experienced a miscarriage or stillbirth, being told that this event is a part of God's timing must be devastating. In a cycle of hope/despair after an unsuccessful IVF or repeated unsuccessful attempts to achieve pregnancy, this is crushing. Just how long must we wait (particularly as women often feel the limits of their own fertility in terms of time)? Not only that, but how do we know that attempting to conceive (through intercourse or reproductive technologies) are within the framework of God's timing? And if we are outside those boundaries of God's timing, what will be the results?

The third and final sovereignty myth expresses that through reproductive loss (suffering) God teaches, tests, and seeks to develop character. I once read a Facebook status update written by a woman who recently had experienced a miscarriage that said she knew/hoped that God was teaching her through this experience. This is not to say that we are incapable of discovering something about ourselves or about God, faith, or the Christian community in the midst of experiences of reproductive difficulty and loss. The problem, however, is when that heuristic process transforms into God's active intentions to teach, test our faith, or develop character through the grief and losses associated with reproductive loss. Again, the kind of God who operates in this way is cruel and malevolently manipulative.

No matter what local theologies or theological worldviews a pastor strategically develops within a community of care (inside and outside contexts of congregational worship), I want to unequivocally state that pastors *must* actively respond to these hurtful popular theological formulations. These sovereignty myths damage faith and promote problematic concepts of who God is and what God does in the world. I wonder how long a person can express faith in and faithfulness to a God who acts like this.

As such, it is part of pastoral responsibility to develop in preaching and worship a kind of theologically sophisticated public that actively differentiates between the God of sovereignty myths and the God who wills no one to suffer. If the pastor develops a notion of sovereignty within congregational worldview, then the pastor will need to address the extent and characteristics of God's sovereignty. Pastors will want to carefully develop their theological statements about the role of God in human affairs, particularly our physical bodies, in preaching and worship.[56]

I want to share one final word on pop theology. Although I never heard anyone say this to me, and despite my theological

---

56 This relates, of course, to illness and disability.

training, I raised an internal question trying to explain why we were experiencing reproductive difficulty and loss. I do not think that I am the only one to have asked it: "Is this suffering punishment for past sin?" Pastors, in no uncertain terms, will want to counter the idea that this kind of suffering is punishment for sin. While some of our poorest life(style) choices might have some effects on fertility, God's graceful nature does not in any way inflict punishment on humans in this way.

A sermon or sermon series exploring the concept of God's will should certainly be among the choices for how pastors will address pop theology. There are some creative options here, including framing these questions specifically as listener-generated questions that the pastor willingly addresses. Moments in worship can easily coordinate with the themes raised in preaching, with the goal of preaching and worship supporting one another.

By addressing these specific pastoral and prophetic dimensions, pastors will be engaging multiple dimensions of work toward healing, wholeness, restoration, and the development of a community of care. Since the bulk of the focus has been on discursive practices in congregational worship, most especially preaching, I now turn to think creatively about how we might construct corporate and private rituals that address the previous issues in both non-discursive (symbolic) and discursive ways.

The Pastoral Function of Ritual and Liturgy: Corporate and Private Worship

Christian worship can serve a powerful pastoral function with reproductive loss in view. When worship attempts to address the widest range of human experience, people can find their experience merges with the Divine towards the kind of meaning-making and healing that they desire. Susan White is correct in saying

> Christian worship is an indispensable part of the total pastoral care of men, women, and children at significant moments in their lives. To ritualize joy and grief, to celebrate and

renew commitment, to pray for those embarking on a new
course in life are not only critical factors in the well-being and
psycho-social integration of individuals, but also necessary for
the health of the Christian community as a whole. In all cases,
the longing of human beings to see their lives as having real
meaning is met by the proclamation of the gospel of God's
love for us all, and by a vision of the Christian vocation that
embraces all states of life.[57]

This is a dense definition for the role of worship as pastoral
care. In finding ways to responsibly incorporate experiences of reproductive loss into the church's worship (whether corporate or
private) pastors will attempt to provide rituals that express grief,
mark dreams deferred, and indicate new directions in life. White
also points to worship as important for both individual and communal health when providing care in the context of worship. In
the final sentence of the definition above, she describes the need
for meaning-making, for affirmation of God's enduring love, and
for a sense of vocation (we might also say "call" or "purpose") for
the various experiences and stations of life. These are vital functions
for worship, especially with reproductive loss in view.

Pastors would do well to begin developing ritual frameworks
(meaning flexible ritual activities) for congregants who experience
reproductive loss. Since ritual often has a bad reputation as repet-
itive action void of emotional depth and meaning, a brief word
on the role and power of ritual is in order. In an overly simplistic
definition, rituals are repeated and repeatable actions that both
structure reality and attempt to make sense of reality. We might
consider baptism and Eucharist as two of the main Christian rituals.
In this sense, rituals attempt to embody and enact ideas (on which
we have largely focused to this point) as much as ideas are shaped
by ritual practices. Catherine Bell points to different categories of
ritual: rites of passage; calendrical and commemorative rites; rites
of exchange and communion; rites of affliction; rites of feasting,

---

57 Susan J. White, *Foundations of Christian Worship*, 1st U.S. ed. (Louisville,
KY: Westminster John Knox Press, 2006), 150-51.

fasting, and festivals; and political rituals.[58] Rites of affliction will often be the focus when reproductive loss is in view. According to Bell, "rituals of affliction attempt to rectify a state of affairs that has been disturbed or disordered; they heal, exorcise, protect, and purify...[T]he dynamics of the ritual attempt to redress the development of anomalies or imbalances."[59] For those attempting to move past reproductive loss, whether through pursuing adoption or abandoning attempts for children altogether, rites of passage will be more appropriate.

Herbert Anderson and Edward Foley write about the significant function of ritual for religious meaning-making. They contend that "rituals are essential and powerful means for making the world an habitable and hospitable place. They are a basic vehicle for creating and expressing meaning. They are an indispensable medium by which we make our way through life."[60] They go on to connect ritual to the human impulse to use narrative as a way of making meaning. Rituals, whether passed on for generations, or constructed for new situations, help people to move from one state in life to another and enable us to make sense of our experiences. They are "imaginative and interpretive act[s] through which we express and create meaning in our lives."[61]

The bottom line for worship and ritual is this: liturgy that intentionally shapes ritual action functions as means by which communities of faith enable each other to interpret life's varied experiences and order the accompanying narratives in a meaningful way. As such, ritual can be a powerful liturgical tool for helping make sense of reproductive loss, express one's story, and find the means to incorporate that narrative into the larger framework of faith.

---

58 Catherine M. Bell, *Ritual: Perspectives and Dimensions* (New York: Oxford University Press, 1997), 94.

59 Ibid., 115.

60 Herbert Anderson and Edward Foley, *Mighty Stories, Dangerous Rituals: Weaving Together the Human and the Divine*, 1st ed. (San Francisco: Jossey-Bass, 1998), 22.

61 Ibid., 26.

The example rituals I suggest below are certainly not exhaustive. The contours of specific rituals will vary according to what local theologies and theological worldviews the pastor thinks is valuable (both weekly and long-term), in addition to the unique situations encountered among the congregation.

CORPORATE RITUALS SURROUNDING REPRODUCTIVE LOSS

In terms of corporate rituals, begin by examining each moment in a congregational liturgy for potential moments for healing, wholeness, restoration, and the development of a community of care. Develop rituals that operate within the framework of regular weekly congregational worship and incorporate the pastoral and prophetic tasks outlined above. While there are prayers in some denominational worship books for miscarriages and/or stillbirths, the worship resources for the wider range of reproductive losses are fewer, and will best be developed on the ground as pastors and congregations find ways to respond that best fit their context. The specific practices will vary among different traditions and according to different theological responses to these losses, but the fourfold structure of worship might provide an imaginative framework for what congregations might do in their liturgies: (1) the people gather, (2) the people listen to God's word, (3) the people respond to God's word heard and proclaimed, and (4) the people depart for service.

In the section of gathering, a prayer of confession might be developed that includes confessing the ways that we have tried to answer people's suffering too easily, with unhelpful thoughts about God's will and timing. Over time, a pastor might work with a worship team and congregational leaders to "train" congregants not to ask individuals if they have children, unless it is obvious they do, during the exchange of the "Peace of Christ." Here is an opportunity to teach/emphasize the Hebrew counterpart "shalom," which we have lifted up as wholeness to the Greek greeting of "peace."

Part of extending the peace to others is extending to them a sense of wholeness, not taking a chance that they will feel their loss afresh just by a greeting, however innocent.

During the section of response,[62] one ritual I suggest relates to the cycles of hope/despair and grief/loss. In the setting of worship, roughly under the moments in the structure of worship classified "response," the pastor might provide the congregation with paper or sticky notes and invite congregants to write on one a hope they have and on another, what precipitates their despair. Similarly, responses could be invited in terms of grief/loss, being mindful to communicate openness toward different kinds of loss (in essence, giving permission for individuals to express their loss). After an ample opportunity for the congregation to record their thoughts, a number of possibilities exist for what to do with them: (1) Invite congregants to keep them and pray over them; (2) in congregational settings where high levels of trust and intimacy exist, invite congregants to share them with someone if they are comfortable; (3) collect them along with the day's tithes/offerings, communicating that God wants us to offer both our strengths and the places where we need to receive God's comfort; (4) or invite congregants to carry what they have written to the altar, cross, or other major liturgical furniture/symbol, communicating God's desire to walk with us in our hope/despair and God's willingness to accept our concerns.

Another possibility involves simply being intentional in a pastoral prayer (or incorporating one if such a prayer does not exist). I suggest lifting up specific themes that I have traced above, being as plain as possible. In addressing God or blessing God, the pastor could express the goodness of God, the knowledge that God does not will our suffering, or the assurance that God does not use our suffering to test us. In thanking God, express gratitude for the multiple ways that God blesses the different ways that we form and

---

62 I assume that we have sufficiently covered the portion of worship generally called listening or hearing, during which a sermon is normally preached.

act as families. In moments of intercession, pray for fertility clinics, fertility and OBGYN doctors and nurses, and for potential and current patients. Pray for the wisdom and discernment of those trying to decide how they will address their reproductive difficulties/loss. Pray for those whose hopes have been damaged and are grieving the losses of dreams as well as physical realities of pregnancy loss.

Finally, in the section of departing, the pastor can be intentional about structuring benedictions and charges to the congregation. Assure the congregation that though they exit the worship space into a world that can be full of disappointment, God is with them, God is active, and God is creating anew in the world (though the pastor might be careful in language around God "giving birth" to something new). Charge the congregation to be agents of healing, wholeness, and restoration in the world.

Recently, some congregations have begun to offer special worship services to memorialize infant and pregnancy loss, typically in October, which is National Pregnancy and Infant Loss Awareness month.[63] These infant and pregnancy loss services are commendable and offer safe spaces for grief support, care, and meaning-making.

PRIVATE RITUALS SURROUNDING REPRODUCTIVE LOSS

Private rituals allow a different way to process hope, despair, grief, loss, as well as a way to grapple with difficult theological issues.

Serene Jones describes a ritual performed with Wendy, her close friend who has experienced a miscarriage. As they turn over dirt in the rain and bury some of the collected remnants of Wendy's pregnancy, this burial ritual provides a way of marking in time grief and loss. In Bell's terms, this would be a ritual of passage (death) and of affliction. For those who are unable to achieve a pregnancy and are transitioning from that reality to another, I might suggest a similar kind of burial. Individuals or couples could write down

63 See http://www.october15th.com.

the hopes and dreams that were part of their vision for a biological pregnancy: emotions and feelings, hoped-for biological experiences, and any "artifacts" from the fertility journey with which they are willing to part. In situations where the pastoral relationship is strong, the pastor could accompany the burial for prayer or just to provide pastoral presence as that burial takes place.

In situations where pastors are privileged to know these situations, they might pray with individuals or couples before fertility treatments/procedures or provide a prayer guide which helps lead individuals or couples in pray on their own before, during periods of waiting, and on occasions of success or failure.[64] An additional step would be to provide times and spaces in a congregation's sacred space for individuals or couples to express their narratives, their fears, and/or their hopes (perhaps as with an infant and pregnancy loss service). Writing, lighting candles, and specific places and postures of prayer might be especially useful.

Having addressed major issues around preaching and worship as they related to reproductive loss, our attention can now shift to preaching and worship with adoption in view.

---

64 I have included such resources in the supplementary materials.

Chapter Three

Constructing a Theology of Adoption for Preaching and Worship

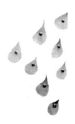

Each year in the United States approximately 120,000 children are adopted through domestic and international adoptions.[65] The hope is to create "forever families," (a preferred adoption terminology) by which parent(s) and children form a relationship of mutual care and nurture. As opposed to even twenty-five years ago, adoption has taken on a radically different public image. With the rise of "open" domestic adoptions (where one or both birthparents and adoptive families have some level of contact with one another) and the increase in international (otherwise known as intercountry or transnational) adoptions, the public is much more informed about adoption. Many of the stigmas and stereotypes attached to adoptive children, adoptive parents, and even to great extent, birthparents of adopted children have waned. The "adoption triad," those immediately aforementioned parties, coexist in much different ways than they have in the past. The pressure to hide or minimize the realities of adoption has diminished among many of the families and larger networks of those who come into contact with the adoption triad.

Even with these changes, the decision to adopt has many different faces. Decisions about how a family will be formed are unique to each situation. Some will have success with assisted reproductive technologies, and while considerations for adoption may have been on the table at one time, now they are removed. Other times, even after biological children come along, some decide to adopt. The

---

65 "Facts for Families: The Adopted Child," American Academy of Child and Adolescent Psychiatry, http://www.aacap.org/AACAP/ Families_and_Youth/Facts_for_Families/Facts_for_Families_Pages/The_ Adopted_Child_15.aspx.

presence of biological and adopted children are not always mutually exclusive in a family. Certainly after the difficulties of assisted reproductive technologies, some will end their attempts to children for any number of reasons. Adoption may or may not have ever been a realistic possibility for them. For some, adoption will be a first step, bypassing attempts at biological children altogether, without having experienced a kind of biological reproductive loss at all. Some adoptions will occur through family mergers and other circumstances. From foster adoptions to domestic and international adoptions, each choice to adopt has a unique set of circumstances and unique processes that accompany them. This is not to mention both the fear of and occurrences of failed or ruptured adoptions, which dematerialize due to their own unique circumstances, and present their own sense of loss.

Since the early 2000s, adoption has received an increased profile among faith communities, and particularly in Christian communities. Adoptions that have occurred in North American celebrity culture have, no doubt, contributed to that raised profile and access to information about adoption. Movies like *Juno* (2007) brought adoption into the spotlight on the big screen. The stigmas once associated with the adoption process, adoptive parents, children, and biological parents continue to fall by the wayside. As constituents of adoption triads move into the mainstream and tell their stories, adoption has come out from the shadows of misunderstanding.

Many so-called Evangelical communities have articulated a biblical mandate to "care for orphans." The phenomenon has been articulated by Evangelical leaders like Rick Warren and spread throughout publications such as *Christianity Today*, large conferences, and trickles down to Evangelical pulpits. The editor's notes section of the July 2010 issue of *Christianity Today* proclaims in its headline, "Adoption is Everywhere: Even God is into it."[66] In these notes, Ted Olsen, managing editor for news and online journalism

---

66   Ted Olsen, "Adoption Is Everywhere: Even God Is into It," *Christianity Today* 54, no. 7 (2010): 5.

draws attention to the December 2009 issue, in which adoption
was number six on a list of "Top Ten Theology Stories of 2009."
The organization Together for Adoption identifies its mission as
"providing gospel-centered resources to mobilize the church for
global orphan care."[67] A similar organization called the Christian
Alliance for Orphans (CAFO) outlines its work: "As the Alliance
helps Christians understand God's call to care for the orphan and
equips them for effective response, the impact reaches far beyond
a single program or met need. Rather, an ever-expanding army of
passionate advocates invest time, talent and treasure in a *personal* and *sustained commitment* to caring for orphans in the name of
Christ."[68] In identifying these groups, Olsen also points to Evangelicals "who, faced with the seemingly countless ways to pursue
social justice and compassion, are starting with the 'orphans and
widows' of James 1:27. Other friends praise the focus on adoption
for being an important family issue that sidesteps the ceaseless
debates on 'gay stuff.' Then again, other friends see adoption as
the new battleground over homosexuality."[69] In that statement,
Olsen identifies how adoption correlates to wider discussions in
Evangelical subculture.[70]

In this case a wide range of issues converge to make adoption
an issue for Evangelicals. The cover story from that 2010 issue
of *Christianity Today*, is entitled "Abba changes Everything: Why
Every Christian is Called to Rescue Orphans."[71] In it, Russell D.
Moore suggests that

---

67 "Home Page," Together for Adoption, http://www.togetherforadoption.
    org.
68 "Core Principles," Christian Alliance for Orphans, http://www.aacap.org/
    AACAP/Families_and_Youth/Facts_for_Families/Facts_for_Families_
    Pages/The_Adopted_Child_15.aspx.
69 Olsen, "Adoption Is Everywhere: Even God Is into It," 5.
70 Interestingly, the quote from both CAFO and Olsen use "battle"
    language to describe the issues surrounding the church and adoption.
71 Russell D. Moore, "Abba Changes Everything: Why Every Christian Is
    Called to Rescue Orphans," *Christianity Today* 54, no. 7 (2010).

Adoption is, on one hand, gospel. Our identity and inheritance are grounded in our adoption in Christ. Adoption
is also *mission*. In this, our adoption spurs us to join Christ
in advocating for the poor, the marginalized, the abandoned,
and the fatherless. Without the theological aspect, the growing
Christian emphasis on orphan care too often seems like one
more cause wristband for compassionate conservative evangelicals to wear until the trend dies down. Without the missional
aspect, the doctrine of adoption too easily becomes mere metaphor, just another way to say 'saved.'[72]

A deep connection to a doctrine of salvation, a thriving idea of
mission, biblical literalism, concern for the family, a commitment
to ending abortion, concerns over homosexuality, and renewed
concerns for social justice have affected a tremendous rise in the
number of adoptions in the Evangelical community. In fact, these
convergent issues seem to have formed an ethical imperative for
many who are part of this aspect of North American Christianity.

However, this raised and public profile has not necessarily
been the case among so-called mainline Protestants.[73] As with reproductive difficulty and loss, there has been silence and avoidance
in preaching and worship. This chapter and the next are devoted to
similar tasks as those discussed regarding reproductive loss: overcoming silence and avoiding avoidance in congregational worship
as it relates to adoption.

If we are going to preach and worship in ways that overcome
silence and avoid avoidance, we will need to return once again
to the biblical texts from which most sermons have their starting point. And in the case of adoption, this is a felicitous task.
Rather than "texts of terror" presenting a problem in need of a
sensitive reading and reconstruction, here in the case of adoption
there are some powerful individual stories that open up adoption
as a positive, divinely-inspired familial occurrence. Even more, the

---

72 Ibid., 20.

73 In this case, I think there are some things mainline Protestants, who are
    often averse to learning from Evangelicals, have much to receive, even
    with the critiques mainline Protestants would return.

metaphor of adoption in the New Testament initiates a powerful picture of the persons of the Trinity, their relationship to one another (even amid historical, doctrinal controversy), and the nature of salvation. In what follows below, I will (1) trace these texts as well as the images of God they convey, then (2) summarize how these texts and images work together to build a biblical theology of adoption with practical theological import.

ADOPTION IN THE BIBLE

Adoptive Relationships in the Old Testament/ Hebrew Bible

There remains some disagreement as to how exactly (and to some degree, if) the practice of adoption existed in the Ancient Near East, and more specifically, if it was practiced legally among the Israelite people of the Old Testament.[74] We should not be surprised that adoption did not take the same sort of legal and functional shape that it does now. Even so, the exact legality and procedures of adoption in the Ancient Near East have little bearing on the reality that throughout time, men and women have in some way claimed children not born to them biologically as their sons and daughters. Regardless of the procedure or technical term assigned to the practices of what we would call adoption, the Hebrew Bible contains stories of several figures we can identify as living in adoptive relationships.

Some of the characters and their stories are familiar territory. The story of the exodus of the Hebrew people has its origins in Pharaoh's decree that the male Hebrew children be killed by throwing each newborn male in the Nile River. After his birth, Moses'

74 The technicality of these arguments and the historical origins/practice of adoption in the Ancient Near East is best left outside the purview of this book. For more depth, see: Meir Malul, "Adoption of Foundlings in the Bible and Mesopotamian Documents: A Study of Some Legal Metaphors in Ezekiel 16:1-7," *Journal for the Study of the Old Testament*, no. 46 (1990).

biological mother hid Moses for three months, then made a plan to see if he might be claimed. It is Pharaoh's own daughter who, coming to the river to bathe, sees the child in the basket. While Moses' sister makes a way for Moses' biological mother to nurse the child, Exodus 2:10 completes the story of Moses' adoption: "When the child grew up, she [Moses' biological mother, who was nursing him] brought him to Pharaoh's daughter, and she took him as her son. She named him Moses, 'because,' she said, 'I drew him out of the water.'" The beginning of the Hebrew liberation narrative begins with a clever birth mother and an adoption story.

Samuel's narrative is quite different. Hannah, of course, had experienced reproductive difficulty and she had promised any male child born to her as a servant to God (1 Samuel 1:11). After Samuel is born and Hannah has completed his weaning,

> She took him up with her [to Shiloh], along with a three-year-old bull, an ephah of flour, and a skin of wine. She brought him to the house of the Lord at Shiloh; and the child was young. Then they slaughtered the bull, and they brought the child to Eli. And she said, 'Oh, my lord! As you live, my lord, I am the woman who was standing here in your presence, praying to the Lord. For this child I prayed; and the Lord has granted me the petition that I made to him. Therefore I have lent him to the Lord; as long as he lives, he is given to the Lord.' She left him there for the Lord. (1 Samuel 1:24-28)

Samuel came under the care of the priest Eli and grew up with him until his death. The relationship between Hannah, Samuel, and Eli might be called a type of "open adoption." Hannah is never fully out of contact with Samuel, bringing him a handmade robe every year when she returned to Shiloh to offer her yearly sacrifice (1 Samuel 1:19). Samuel becomes the one who is the mouthpiece of God for Israel and the one who oversees the establishment of Israel's monarchy.

Finally, the Jewish festival of Purim, a celebration of deliverance, has its origins in the narrative of Esther. According to the book bearing her name, "Mordecai had brought up Hadassah, that is Esther, his cousin, for she had neither father nor mother; the girl was fair and beautiful, and when her father and her mother died, Mordecai adopted her as his own daughter" (Esther 2:7). When Esther wins what amounts to a beauty contest held by King Ahasuerus, the king of Persia, she is able to outwit a man named Haman, who wished to annihilate the Jews. Not only does she outwit Haman and avert the slaughter of her people, she also wins favor for them and for Mordecai. As with Moses and the Exodus, the deliverance of God's people takes place through the course of an adoptive relationship.

There are stories that may be less familiar, even with well-known characters. Near the end of the Jacob and Joseph saga in Genesis, Jacob lies on his bed ill and preparing for death. Joseph returns from Egypt to visit him, bringing with him his two sons Ephraim and Manasseh. As Joseph arrives and consults with his father, Jacob makes this promise:

> God Almighty appeared to me at Luz in the land of Canaan, and he blessed me, and said to me, 'I am going to make you fruitful and increase your numbers; I will make of you a company of peoples, and will give this land to your offspring after you for a perpetual holding.' Therefore your two sons, who were born to you in the land of Egypt before I came to you in Egypt, are now mine; Ephraim and Manasseh shall be mine, just as Reuben and Simeon are. As for the offspring born to you after them, they shall be yours. They shall be recorded under the names of their brothers with regard to their inheritance. (Genesis 48:3-6)

While this does not seem like a contemporary adoption for the purposes of meeting the desire for children within a family, Jacob claims Ephraim and Manasseh, his grandsons, and places them on equal footing as his own sons with regard to their inheritance. Jacob "adopts" Ephraim and Manasseh for the purposes of blessing them and fully including them into the family line.

Similarly, in Genesis 15 Abram speaks with God about God's promise and his childlessness. Again, though not technically what we might consider an adoptive relationship for the same purposes as contemporary ones, Abram identifies Eliezer of Damascus as his heir, "a slave born in my house" (Genesis 15:3). Nowhere does Abram identify Eliezer as his son, but as with Jacob, the concern for the continuation of family and the transfer of family inheritance is an important factor. For Abram, it is important enough to designate someone outside his own bloodline to carry forward what Abram will pass on, though as his conversation with God suggests, Abram is not happy that this has to be the case.

Still, many of these characters are unfamiliar to many readers and their stories are quite brief. Another relationship found in the pages of the Hebrew Bible might stretch our concept of adoption. Judges 11 outlines the origins of Jephthah, who was "the son of a prostitute," born to Gilead. Jephthah lived in Gilead's house along with Gilead's wife and the sons born to her. Jephthah was driven out of the house by the sons of Gilead's wife (a kind of adoptive mother) when they told him, "You shall not inherit anything in our father's house; for you are the son of another woman" (Judges 11:2). This situation shows the tenuousness of adoptive relationships in the Ancient Near East (even if, technically, we do not see adoption here in the contemporary form) and the tie between adoption and inheritance, as with Ephraim, Manasseh, and Eliezer.

1 Kings details the character Hadad, who was a survivor of Joab's slaughter of the male Edomites. As a young boy, Hadad fled to Egypt and was taken in by the pharaoh, "who gave him a house, assigned him an allowance of food, and gave him land" (1 Kings 11:18). Hadad developed a trusted relationship with the pharaoh, who also gave him his sister-in-law (the queen's sister) as his wife. Hadad's wife bore him a son, whom he gave the name Genubath. Genubath was weaned by Tahpenes, the pharaoh's wife, and was raised with the rest of the pharaoh's children in the pharaoh's household. Here we might say we see a kind of "open adoption," where though raised in a different household, (we suppose) Genubath had access to his birth family.

Finally, in these briefer stories, we see the story of Obed. Obed was born to Ruth and Boaz. The narrator of the book of Ruth emphasizes the importance of Obed to Naomi, Ruth's mother-in-law. The women surrounding Naomi proclaim God's blessing on Naomi through Obed and the narrator records how Naomi "took the child and laid him in her bosom, and became his nurse. The women of the neighborhood gave him a name, saying, 'A son has been born to Naomi.' They named him Obed" (Ruth 4:16-17). Though we will not want to press an adoptive relationship too far here, it is important to note that Naomi becomes a caretaker for Obed and the neighborhood women identify Obed as Naomi's son, even if not in a literal sense.

What are we to make of these characters and their relationships? Mary Foskett helpfully reminds us that in Moses' case, it cannot be overlooked that from the perspective of Moses the adoptee, his identity was contested from an early point in his career.[75] Was he an Egyptian or one of the Hebrew people, or somehow belonging to both groups at once? The negotiation of this identity has everything to do with what happened with Moses' birth narrative and his "adoption" into Pharaoh's household. Along with adoption comes a complex understanding of one's identity and the process for sorting through that identity is unique in each instance. We can imagine the difficulty Moses might have had in being both Egyptian and one of the few Hebrew boys his age to survive Pharaoh's slaughter. The same would apply for Genubath and, though not a culturally conflicted identity, certainly Jephthah's story is one of intra-familial conflict, being born to a prostitute yet living in his father's household with siblings born to another woman. The adoptive relationships in the Hebrew Bible point to the complexity of identity construction for the adoptee.

More obvious is the fact that these names and their stories are preserved as a record of people of note in the religious histo-

---

75 Mary F. Foskett, "The Accidents of Being and the Politics of Identity: Biblical Images of Adoption and Asian Adoptees in America," *Semeia*, no. 90-91 (2002).

ry of ancient Israel. From these characters come the narratives of God's presence and protection for the people of Israel. Ephraim and Manasseh, Moses, Samuel, and Esther in particular move the people of Israel into deeper covenant relationship with God. Inasmuch as the Old Testament details a salvation history of the people of Israel, adoptive relationships play key roles in moving along the narrative of God's liberating, salvific activity among God's chosen people. God's work in and among humanity does not come solely through biological familial relationships, but through multiple constructions of family.

Orphan Care in the Old Testament/Hebrew Bible

In addition to the stories that outline adoptive-type relationships, we should note the overwhelming directive from the Old Testament to care for orphans. This directive does not prescribe adoption in either ancient or contemporary forms. There are close to fifty references to orphans in the Old Testament books (most often directly connected with widows). The overwhelming number of those references instruct God's people to extend justice to orphans, to not abuse orphans, to include them in the promises of God's people, to allow them to glean from the harvest, to include them in the tithe, and to defend them from oppression. These directives take the form of commands in Exodus, Deuteronomy, and Proverbs as well as accusations against God's people for their failure to do so in the Prophetic books (Isaiah, Jeremiah, Ezekiel, Hosea, Zechariah, Malachi). Job questions God, in part, on the basis of those who seem to flourish while harming the orphan (Job 24:3, 9). Job also defends his righteousness by the example of his care for orphans (29:12; 31:18). In the Psalms, God is identified as the helper of orphans (10:14), the Father of orphans (68:5), and the one who watches over orphans (146:9).

Repeatedly, God implores God's people to provide for those who have no care and no protection from birthparents. For this vulnerable group of people, God seems to be especially concerned.

God's people are judged by how they care for orphans (in addition to widows and aliens) and failure to extend justice or life-giving attention results in breach of the covenant God has extended. In short, care of the orphan should be a hallmark of God's people, according to the Old Testament witness.

Adoption in the New Testament

As we move into the New Testament, the focus shifts. We do not see the same types of narratives or characters as we saw in the Hebrew Bible. There are, however, two distinct foci as we consider adoption: (1) the person and status of Jesus as son and (2) the metaphor of God as adoptive parent as used by the Apostle Paul in regard to people of faith.

Before launching into these two foci, a brief word on the role of adoption in the Greco-Roman world is in order. Adoption in the time of Jesus and the first Christians, by and large, did not take place out of the experiences of childlessness, at least not as we might experience it today. Instead, adoptions were performed out of concern for legal transfer of property and inheritances (similar to the case of Abram in Genesis). Adoptees were already (mostly male) adults and adoption (by male property-holders) was executed to transfer privileges and new responsibilities to the adoptee. Of course, this will color our understanding of how adoption is used in the New Testament literature as the transfer of inheritance. It does not, however, prevent adoption from serving as a rich metaphor.

Jesus as Adopted?

How does Jesus relate to adoption? This is a thorny question, but an important one. While researching questions surrounding adoption and the New Testament, I engaged social media to ask some church historians and biblical scholars about Jesus as adoptee and in particular the place of Jesus in the development of historical heresy known as "adoptionism." Their response was interesting. The small handful that responded in depth encouraged me to push past Jesus as adoptee and to focus exclusively on Paul's use of adoption as a much more fruitful place to develop thought on adoption. I found this to be a remarkable phenomenon. Something about Jesus as adoptee feels just slightly out of place for those acquainted with, and concerned about, historical theology. Yet those who were guilty of this early heresy found something deeply compelling about the idea of Jesus as adopted son. As an adoptive parent, I find this view of Jesus compelling as well for different reasons, and at least worthy of some reflection.

Briefly, adoptionism has its roots in 8th-century Spanish theologians Felix of Urgel and Elipandus of Toledo, who "held that, while the Second Person of the Trinity is eternal, the man Jesus was adopted as God's son through grace."[76] Justo Gonzalez notes that "more commonly, the term 'adoptionism' is used to refer to any doctrine that holds that Jesus was a man whom God adopted into sonship. Thus, the Ebionites and many Antiochene theologians of the fourth and fifth centuries are sometimes called adoptionists. For similar reasons, some accuse nineteenth century liberal theology of having adoptionistic tendencies."[77] In short, adoptionism focuses on the human Jesus, whose relationship to God changes/increases through the course of his life, "based upon the gradual development of Jesus' consciousness" (most notably in his baptism).[78]

We recognize that the adoptionist stance denigrates the human-divine Jesus in favor of a more human conception of Jesus who eventually grows into his divinity, either by earning it or developing it.[79] Still, it does present a picture of Jesus as adoptee with

---

76 Justo L. González, *Essential Theological Terms*, 1st ed. (Louisville, KY: Westminster John Knox Press, 2005), 2. I do not consider the "son of God" references in the Gospels as adoptionist links, since historical Jesus research has shown this saying to have specific meaning in the context of Jewish history.

77 Ibid.

78 Thomas C. Oden, *The Word of Life*, 1st ed. (San Francisco: Harper & Row, 1989), 241.

79 Ibid., 242.

which other adoptees might identify. This act of heresy (even if a momentary chance for reflection) provides positive ground for the difficult work of sifting through issues of identity, particularly with persistent negative associations about adoption in the culture at-large. For instance, the adoptee might ask: "If Jesus was adopted, what might that say about me? How is it that I identify with Jesus the adoptee? What might that say about adoption?" Such questions position Jesus as adoptee *par excellence* and a mediator of adoptive identity.

Furthermore, how do we picture Joseph? Is he also an adoptive father (and does he stand alone as adoptive father or somehow in conjunction with the First Person of the Trinity)? Anecdotally speaking, I have heard this description of Joseph from others in conversation. This is more in keeping with a traditional reading of the gospels. If Joseph functions this way, what does this mean for adoptive parents?[80] From a different angle, if an adoptionist Jesus is somehow "less-than" an orthodox Jesus (which is what it felt like when those I consulted encouraged me to look past the adoptionist controversies), we might wonder what that says about the cultural and historical moorings of orthodox theology. Do orthodox versions of theology fear a Jesus who is not "biologically" related to the First Person of the Trinity ("of the same substance," to use language from historical theology)? The history of Christian doctrine certainly responds with a resounding "yes" to that question. These are questions the adoption triad might put to historical theological formulations as they sift through issues of identity, adoption, and theology.

Adoption in the Letters of the New Testament

While adoptionism may be a heretical stance, the images of God as adoptive parent developed by Paul present a deeply mov-

---

80 See Yigal Levin, "Jesus, 'Son of God' and 'Son of David': The 'Adoption' of Jesus into the Davidic Line," *Journal for the Study of the New Testament* 28, no. 4 (2006).

ing image of God's care and concern for humanity. In fact, the images Paul uses of God as adoptive parent are some of the most well developed metaphors in the Pauline corpus to describe God's relationship to humankind.

Before exploring the New Testament texts in detail, a word is in order about the use of the word "adoption" in English translations of the New Testament. The Greek word used in the Pauline passages is *huiothesia* (υἱοθεσία), a compound word consisting of a combination of "son" – *huios* (υἱός) and "to fix or establish" – *tithemi* (τίθημι). As a compound word with clear roots, this is fairly straightforward in terms of what it communicates: a person or people are established/fixed as a child/children of someone else. Frances Lyall believes Paul's use of this term stems from the Roman legal system, which he and the recipients of his letters would certainly know. In this system "the adoptee is taken out of his previous state and is placed in a new relationship with his new *paterfamilias*. All his old debts are canceled, and in effect he starts a new life. From that time the *paterfamilias* owns all the property and acquisitions of the adoptee, controls his personal relationships, and has rights of discipline. On the other hand, he is involved in liability by the actions of the adoptee and owes reciprocal duties of support and maintenance."[81] Here we can begin to see the seeds of what Paul suggests about soteriology through the use of this metaphor.

Paul's fullest use of adoption comes in the theologically dense eighth chapter of Romans, where Paul discusses the relationship between living by the law and the Spirit. Verses 14-16 say, "For all who are led by the Spirit of God are children of God. For you did not receive a spirit of slavery to fall back into fear, but you have received a spirit of adoption. When we cry, 'Abba! Father!' it is that very Spirit bearing witness with our spirit that we are children of God, and if children, then heirs, heirs of God and joint heirs with Christ—if, in fact, we suffer with him so that we may also be glorified with him." Paul speaks of the Spirit as that which provides

---

81   Francis Lyall, "Roman Law in the Writings of Paul: Adoption," *Journal of Biblical Literature* 88, no. 4 (1969): 466.

confirmation of the promise that those who find their lives rooted in Christ are indeed adopted children of God, complete with the inheritance God provides God's children. Paul uses adoption to convey a depth of meaning to the church in Rome. Regarding this extensive exploration of adoption in Romans, Elisabeth Ann Johnson writes that "Paul assures his readers that although we struggle in a world of sin and death, we have not been abandoned to lives of slavery and fear. In Christ, God has claimed us, adopted us as his very own children and heirs. This we know because his Spirit bears witness with our own when we cry out to God."[82]

Continuing this line of thought, Paul says "We know that the whole creation has been groaning in labor pains until now; and not only the creation, but we ourselves, who have the first fruits of the Spirit, groan inwardly while we wait for adoption, the redemption of our bodies. For in hope we were saved. Now hope that is seen is not hope. For who hopes for what is seen? But if we hope for what we do not see, we wait for it with patience" (8:22-24). Again, adoption is used within the context of salvation and, oddly enough, mixed with a metaphor about childbirth. In these mixed metaphors Paul seems to make a qualitative difference between the redemption of humans and the rest of creation. Both experience anticipatory groaning, but creation will give birth to something new and humanity, having already been born, will itself be adopted into a new relationship. Here adoption does not simply convey the texture of salvation; instead adoption becomes eschatological in nature.

Further, the waiting described in chapter 8 give a now/not yet picture of redemption that may be familiar to many in the adoptive triad. For instance, in the early days after my wife and I picked up our daughter from the hospital, we had two legal waiting periods for the adoption to become final. We first waited through a period of two weeks in which the birthmother could reconsider her revocation of parental rights and then a six-month period until we could

---

82 Elizabeth A. Johnson, "Waiting for Adoption: Reflections on Romans 8:12-25," *Word & World* 22, no. 3 (2002): 309.

legally finalize our adoption in court (both were state laws). Bringing the scripture and life experience together, Johnson continues,

> the adoption metaphor...helpfully illustrates the reality of our lives as redeemed children of God. The adoption papers have been signed; we have been sealed by the Spirit at baptism. Yet we continue to experience anguish and struggle until the time when that adoption will be complete and we will be truly 'home' with God. In the meantime we often groan in pain and frustration as we experience the inevitable tension between belonging to God and yet living in the world of sin and death and decay.[83]

In other words, salvation as adoption is both a guarantee of a present state and a promissory note of something more (and better) yet to come.

In chapter 9, Paul explores the role of Israel and Paul's frustration with his own people and their relationship to Jesus: "I have great sorrow and unceasing anguish in my heart. For I could wish that I myself were accursed and cut off from Christ for the sake of my own people, my kindred according to the flesh. They are Israelites, and to them belong the adoption, the glory, the covenants, the giving of the law, the worship, and the promises; to them belong the patriarchs, and from them, according to the flesh, comes the Messiah, who is over all, God blessed forever. Amen" (9:2-5). Paul is frustrated that his "own people" do not see the continuing work of God in Jesus, having already received the gift of adoption.

Galatians 4 borrows ideas from the earlier section of Romans 8. As Galatians is written for the context of misunderstanding about the relationship of Jewish Christians to Gentile Christians, Paul seeks to put both groups on level ground as recipients of the work of Jesus. He says,

> My point is this: heirs, as long as they are minors, are no better than slaves, though they are the owners of all the property; but they remain under guardians and trustees until

---

83 Ibid., 311.

the date set by the father. So with us; while we were minors, we were enslaved to the elemental spirits of the world. But when the fullness of time had come, God sent his Son, born of a woman, born under the law, in order to redeem those who were under the law, so that we might receive adoption as children. And because you are children, God has sent the Spirit of his Son into our hearts, crying, 'Abba! Father!' So you are no longer a slave but a child, and if a child then also an heir, through God" (4:1-7).

Again, Paul seeks to outline the benefits of being included in the household of God, an opportunity available for both Jews and Gentiles, and the now/not-yet (eschatological) sense of adoption.

Finally, in the Pauline corpus, Ephesians 1 also explores the metaphor of adoption and the inheritance associated with life in God through Jesus Christ:

Blessed be the God and Father of our Lord Jesus Christ, who has blessed us in Christ with every spiritual blessing in the heavenly places, just as he chose us in Christ before the foundation of the world to be holy and blameless before him in love. He destined us for adoption as his children through Jesus Christ, according to the good pleasure of his will, to the praise of his glorious grace that he freely bestowed on us in the Beloved. In him we have redemption through is blood, the forgiveness of our trespasses, according to the riches of his grace that he lavished on us. With all wisdom and insight he has made known to us the mystery of his will, according to the good pleasure that he set forth in Christ, as a plan or the fullness of time, to gather up all things in him, things in heaven and things on earth. In Christ we have also obtained an inheritance, having been destined according to the purpose of him who accomplishes all things according to his counsel and will, so that we, who were the first to set our hope on Christ, might live for the praise of his glory. In him you also, who you had heard the word of truth, the gospel of your salvation, and had believed in him, were marked with the seal of the promised Holy Spirit; this is the pledge of our inheritance toward redemption as God's own people, to the praise of his glory. (Ephesians 1:3-14)

These words from Paul offer thanksgiving, blessing, and praise to God for the relationship and inheritance given through Jesus. The focus here is not so much on the contours of the adoptive relationship, but rather the inheritance: redemption, forgiveness, lavish grace, and the promise of the Holy Spirit, all in the fullness of time. As we might expect from the Greco-Roman setting, adoption was significant because of the inheritance rights it bestowed on the adoptee. Here Paul communicates the significance of what God gives to humanity through the work of Jesus.

Orphan Care in the Book of James

The book of James carries forward the ethical imperative of the Old Testament in its encouragement of the Christian community to care for orphans: "Religion that is pure and undefiled before God, the Father, is this: to care for orphans and widows in their distress, and to keep oneself unstained by the world" (1:27). Because of the tradition of James' ministry being centered in Jerusalem, we should not be surprised to hear the words of the Torah and Prophets carried forward. That it is one of the ethical imperatives mentioned explicitly by James suggests both its importance to the ethical life of the emerging Jewish-Christian community and the continuity with the Jewish tradition in which the Christian community found its ethical witness. The Christian community stands in line with God's ethical imperative to extend justice and provide care for the vulnerable.

BUILDING A BIBLICAL THEOLOGY OF ADOPTION

With these texts under consideration, it is important to begin piecing together a biblical theology of adoption that can form and inform preaching and worship. In this sense, theological reflection precedes practice in the practical theological loop as we consider what the biblical witness has to say concerning adoption. There are at least six areas in which we can begin building this biblical theology as a foundation for preaching and worship.

»   *Adoption as Agapic Act*

The biblical witness provides images of love that each member of the adoption triad can live into in some way, shape, or form. In the Bible, adoption is not a shameful act to be hidden, nor to regret. Instead adoption is an agapic act on the part of both adoptive parents and birthparents. For birthparents, child relinquishment is not "giving up" a child, as the phrase is often used.[84] Instead, child relinquishment is an act of showing love, of ensuring that a child will be cared for in a way that the birthparent is unable to provide. Additionally, adoptive parents receive adoptive children from birthparents as a kind of gift. Verity A. Jones recognizes that "An adopted child is received as a gift by her new family, just as the adopting family is a gift to the child. In the same way, the spirit of adoption that Paul commends to the reader is one of gift. It is Paul's way of describing the gift God gives to us in Christ."[85] For those who adopt out of reproductive difficulty especially, this is not something adoptive parents could achieve on their own. And adoption is certainly not a type of reciprocal exchange. Though there are fees and high prices to pay on the part of birthparents and adoptive parents, the fundamental act of handing over a child functions outside the market economy to which we are accustomed in other arenas of life (recognizing that illicit, for-profit adoptions do happen). As a result, adoptive children are given and received as an entrusted gift.

---

84   I will revisit the idea of "giving up" a child in a section on adoption-friendly language in chapter four.

85   Verity A. Jones, "Up for Adoption," *Christian Century* 119, no. 14 (2002): 22.

»   *The Adoptive Household of God*

The biblical witness supplies a robust image of God who chooses adoption to freely and lovingly expand God's household. Paul chooses the image of adoption to develop ideas about salvation. God passes along the blessings of God's household to others through adoption. Despite the important feminine imagery, we get of God in places through the biblical witness (and we are indebted to the contributions of feminist biblical scholars and theologians who have gone to great lengths to show us this imagery), God does not expand God's household through childbirth, at least according to Paul. Instead, God functions as benevolent *paterfamilias*, passing along the inheritance to Jews and Gentiles alike, and promising to seal the adoption in the eschaton. Verity Jones reminds us that "If our families of origin invoke pain and suffering in our hearts (our experience of the flesh, as Paul would say), we can be comforted by the knowledge that we are adopted into another family—literally… or spiritually and ultimately, for everyone who becomes a Christian and is redeemed by God in Christ. Whatever our experience of family loss and brokenness, we will always belong to God."[86] Even those who do not experience the bonds of adopted family literally in this life experience them through life in Christ. God loves and saves the world, in the largest sense, through the act of adoption, of bringing the world in close relationship to God's self.

»   *Self-image and Identity*

The portrayal of God as adoptive parent and deity who cares about the welfare of orphans draws out the kind of picture that might help those connected to adoption (specifically the adoption triad and extended families) see God and the self in relation to God through a new lens. For extended families who might be skeptical or ashamed of adoption, birthparents weighing making an adoption plan, or prospective adoptive parents who are having difficulty making the decision to adopt, identifying God as adoptive parent enables these parties to see God and consider their

86 Ibid.

decisions through a positive theological lens. Again, Verity Jones provides helpful insight: "If we say God's love for us is like that of a parent and Christian community is like family, aren't we saying that adoptive relationships are as worthwhile as biological relationships?"[87] Additionally, adoptees who struggle with self-image, identity, and self-worth might be able to see themselves in relation to God, birthparent(s), and/or adoptive parent(s) in a new way through how God is seen in the biblical witness. A god who loves outside biological bloodlines and cares about the welfare of orphans in particular may provide the kind of theological space to see a person's adopted identity in a new way.

» *Biblical Witness as Transitional Space*

Similarly, use of the biblical witness can provide a transitional space from which people can move from the hopes and desires for biological parenthood to adoptive parenthood, if that is the path they choose. For many the choice to move from attempts for biological parenthood to adoptive parenthood is not only emotionally difficult, but requires grounding in a larger framework. A strong biblical theology of adoption can provide the kind of framework by which that transition can be made, at the very least, with some idea of the permission the biblical narratives give for this kind of parenthood. In other words, God is not limited to childbirth for expanding God's own household, but rather enthusiastically expands God's household through adoption. Samuel and Eli's relationship, as well as Mordecai and Esther's relationship provide the kind of narratives by which adoptive parents might see a loving, fruitful adoptive relationship through which God is present and active.

» *Narrative Space for Self-Exploration*

As suggested by Mary Foskett above, the Hebrew Bible narratives might be used to explore contested identities of adoptees. What might it feel like to be Moses, Esther, Genubath, or even Jesus? Birthparents considering making an adoption plan might

---

87 Ibid.

ask what it would have been like for Moses' biological mother to make a plan for his care or for Hannah to entrust Samuel to Eli. Adoptive parents might ask what would it have been like for Pharaoh's daughter to become the parent for Moses or Mordecai to become the parent for Esther. These stories provide a kind of narrative space for self-exploration. Placing ourselves in the shoes of others from wherever we might sit in the adoption triad can prove to be a helpful exercise, even without experience within the adoption triad. This is similar to the idea of providing transitional space, as described above, but the biblical narratives can provide a lifetime of narrative space for revisiting contested identities or exploring feelings, in addition to grounding adoption in the larger story of God and God's people.

»   *Ethical Mandate*

Finally, a biblical theology of adoption and orphan care provides an ethical mandate for the church. For the church, adoption and orphan care is not simply an option for growing one's family. Instead, adoption and orphan care is an integral justice issue for the entire church. Here is where the so-called Evangelical emphasis on orphan care comes into play. A straight-line, literal interpretation of passages like James 1:27 and the Old Testament passages makes it clear that the care of those children whose birthparents are not in the picture lies deep at the center of what it means to respond to God in action. As we see care for orphans throughout the biblical texts, we come to see that this is an issue about which God deeply cares. As a result, people of faith respond to who God is and what God has done in the world by extending care to those who are unable to provide their own care. Similar to how the biblical witness addresses the poor as vulnerable (in both Evangelical and mainline circles), the biblical witness also gives a clear picture about how the people of God are to respond to the orphan. To ignore this mandate is to incur the charges made by the prophets on behalf of God, but to fulfill it, on the other hand, is to embody God's desires for justice.

With some building blocks in place for a working theology of adoption, we can discern the pastoral work of preaching and worship. As the church gathers for worship, this can be a public opportunity for developing and expounding on the rich theological meaning of adoption.

Chapter Four:

The Roles of Preaching and Worship with Regard to Adoption

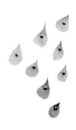

As we bridge from building a more robust theological understanding of adoption to the congregational practices of preaching and worship, it is worth mentioning again that one of the chief tasks of preaching and worship in relationship to adoption is to overcome silence and avoid avoidance. Preaching and worship can help provide moments for framing and re-framing adoption as significant theological events within the life cycle. Intentionally grafting adoption-talk into the liturgical setting creates safe environments in which people can share or contemplate their stories, or paraphrasing Don Saliers, bring their fullest selves to God.[88]

In the Introduction, I outlined some large-scale functions of preaching and worship as they relate to reproductive loss and adoption. These same categories apply when we talk about adoption and while we do not need to completely retrace our steps here, a few words are in order to highlight their application to the contours of adoption rather than reproductive loss. First, the function of "healing and wholeness." If preaching and worship address the physical, emotional, psychological, and spiritual needs of the people who gather together regularly as church, then adoption will also necessarily be part of the range of human experience addressed. The goal (*telos*) of this emphasis will be bringing people to various types of healing from the hurts they experience around adoption as well as encouraging the wholeness of *shalom* in their lives as they await or become accustomed to new family bonds. I will say more about this below in relation to the pastoral tasks of preaching and worship.

---

88 Don E. Saliers, *Worship as Theology: Foretaste of Glory Divine* (Nashville: Abingdon, 1994), 22.

Second, preaching and worship provide opportunities to carry out the task of "theological naming" with regard to adoption. Here it is important to bring to bear the positive message of the biblical witness with regard to adoption and weave it into a constructive local theology with the experiences of those within the horizons of the church community and world. Whatever the contested state of authority preaching and worship have in a wider cultural context, preaching and worship still have the power to frame the world and humans' place within it for those who gather for congregational worship.

Third, with the role of the minister as "guest and host," it is important to note that the minister need not be directly affected by adoption to be able to carry out the work of preaching and planning/leading the congregation's worship. Instead, the minister can listen sensitively and engage as a mutual partner in ministry with the congregation through the tasks of preaching and planning/leading worship. Preaching will be informed by the experiences of the congregation with the intention of hosting ongoing conversation, prayer, and praise that helps those gathered live more faithfully into the emerging theologies of adoption.

Fourth and finally, preaching and worship provide opportunities to establish communities of care and pastoral communication. Here we can envision congregational communities rallying around adoption triads and extended families in moments of crisis and celebration (or at least being exhorted to do so through sermon and liturgy). Preaching and worship can encourage those gathered to engage in "mutuality in ministry, hospitality, and care/compassion for the world."[89] Additionally, as Randall Nichols suggests, preaching and worship can create the kind of "communicative public" that holds adoption and orphan care close to its heart as the people of God, rather than allowing it to linger in the background or worse, remain in silence.

---

89   G. Lee Ramsey, *Care-Full Preaching: From Sermon to Caring Community* (St. Louis, MO: Chalice Press, 2000), 38-51.

PASTORAL AND PROPHETIC TASKS FOR THE WORK OF PREACHING AND WORSHIP

More specifically, when preaching and worship address adoption during the week-to-week gathering of congregations, pastors will have some pastoral and prophetic tasks, in the same way that reproductive loss requires the pastoral and prophetic to be addressed.

Pastoral Tasks

» *Negotiating Decisions and Periods of Waiting*

When thinking about adoption in a congregational context, one of the initial pastoral concerns for adoptive families is the status of being a "waiting family." Once a family unit makes the decision to pursue adoption, it will have to make a number of decisions about which is the most appropriate route to complete the adoption process. There are, of course, several options: domestic (independent/private, agency, foster) or international/intercountry/transnational. Each of these options has its pros and cons depending on the means and desires of the family unit. When a family unit reaches a decision on the route by which they will attempt to adopt, they can begin the process of initiating the adoption. The process is unique for each of these options. Each, however, requires extensive time spent completing paperwork, close work with certified social workers for home studies, and waiting for approvals prior to a child being placed in the home.

One of the preliminary decisions to be made is assessing potential background scenarios of a child and its suitability to the family unit. When I speak with parents who have only ever had experiences with biological children, they are often surprised to hear of the extensive checklist required of adoptive parents in order to make the best match possible between a child and a waiting family. These checklists, which can be several pages long, require significant decisions by the family unit on serious considerations as to what is acceptable to the adoptive family, such as the sex of the child, special needs (of every conceivable type), a child's exposure to drugs/alcohol and the family history of the birthparents. Each family must carefully balance their desires, their financial limitations for care (for instance, of a child with special needs), and their psychological/emotional capacity for family histories, knowing that each decision they make on the checklist might affect how long they will have to wait for a child. For instance, in our family we made the decision that while we did not care about the sex of the child, we could not receive a child placement with various types of mental and physical special needs because we were not able to provide the kind of environment through finances and time to help that child thrive. Other family units will be more or less selective, again, with the important note being that each decision may affect the waiting time for a family.

Waiting times can be long or short, depending on any number of factors. At the time of this writing, intercountry adoptions between the United States and Russia have been discontinued for a little more than a year. Families who were involved in the process and waiting on an adoption from Russia have been stuck in limbo or have had to return to square one to become approved in other countries. At the time our family entered the domestic agency adoption process, we were informed that the wait for an infant placement after completing our paperwork could be anywhere from 1-3 years (thankfully, it took a little less than a year).[90] If a family unit has also had experiences with reproductive loss and experiences with assisted reproductive technologies, there is a possibility of years of waiting and cycles of hope/despair.

All this is to say that waiting can be one of the most pressing and immediate pastoral needs for families who hope to adopt, with uncertainty at the end and a number of weighty decisions and responsibilities in between. Preaching and worship can help waiting

---

90   "Latest Adoption Cost and Wait Time Data: Results from Adoptive Families' 2009-2010 Cost & Timing of Adoption Survey," http://www. adoptivefamilies.com/articles.php?aid=2161.

families (and extended families) by identifying the groaning and waiting of adoption (Romans 8), exploring themes of patience and hope, lifting up God's comforting presence, exhorting the congregational community as a network of prayer and support, and seeking wisdom/discernment for difficult decisions. These themes are obviously not specific to adoption, so they can be addressed in preaching or acts of worship without singling out waiting families. Knowledge of each waiting family's situation and their place in the adoption process can help shape the pastor's preaching and worship planning.

» *Failed/ruptured adoptions*

It is a sad and painful reality, but not all adoption plans work out. Waiting families can be identified by birthparents as potential matches or one of a few possible matches, only to be informed that the birthparent(s) does not want to continue with the plan for any number of reasons. My family experienced two situations of possible adoption plans falling through prior to our successful placement. This is a continuation of being a waiting family, as described above, so it takes tremendous internal resources to manage what feels like a failure along with the hopes and expectations that accompany the hours/days that a possible adoption plan brings. All kinds of questions can crop up in a failed adoption plan without certainty that those questions will be met with answers: Did the birthparent(s) have a change of heart about the entire adoption process and decide to parent the child? Was something wrong with us that we weren't selected and if so, what? What did another adoptive family say/do/look like that they were chosen by the birthparent(s) over us?[91]

Adoptions can fail or rupture for other reasons. Perhaps the most sensationalized and misunderstood kind of rupture is when birthparent(s) reconsider the termination of parental rights after the child is placed in the adoptive parents' home. "Aren't you scared

---

91 I use the plural here, recognizing that individuals complete adoptions as well.

that the mother will take her back?" is a question some adoptive families will face. Domestic agencies and independent/private domestic adoptive representatives do their best to place waiting children in permanent homes, but state laws exist to protect the rights of both birthparents *and* adoptive parents. In Tennessee, for instance, where we completed our domestic adoption, after signing an initial termination of parental rights, the birthparents had a two-week window in which they could change their minds. Again, this is for their protection. With the agency we used, if in their preliminary work they believed that this was a possibility, the agency would make available a temporary foster caretaker for the child. After that two-week window, and in the six months leading up to finalization of the adoption, it would still have been nearly impossible for the birthparents to restore their parental rights. Most states have similar laws for protection of all parties involved. Still, restoration of parental rights does occur, and it can be painful when it does. This may be more common in situations where adoptive families are going through situations where they foster-to-adopt. Child welfare services do their best to protect children and prioritize keeping biological families intact when it seems in the best interests of the children involved, so children can be reunited with their families of origin. It would be good practice for pastors to become familiar with the laws of the states in which they serve.

Though certainly a small percentage, some adoptive families experience the inability to care for the child after he or she is placed in the home. Again, these stories are sensationalized and popularized by the media. Many of us can recall the recent story of the mother who put the Russian-born child she adopted on a plane back to Russia. The mother insisted that the child was so unruly and violent that she could not care for him. It is true that adoptive families can experience difficulty in caring for children who were born with special needs or who developed special needs in their early days/years for lack of proper nurture in orphanages. Families who experience this must often go to tremendous lengths to train themselves on proper care and to provide the most appropriate environments for children to thrive. Still, there are times when adoptions will be ruptured because a family cannot provide the kind of environment needed for the child to thrive.

In these situations of failed plans and ruptured adoptions, the pastoral tasks of preaching and worship are simple: developing a comforting, caring community that stands in solidarity with one another. Preaching and worship should consistently work against the pop theology and "sovereignty myths" that suggest that failed adoption plans are not part of "God's timing" or that ruptured adoptions are "God's plan." Again, the minister need not address these issues specifically to develop a congregational theology that presses back on sovereignty myths and pop theology. In the course of regular preaching, ministers should be developing a foundation that helps resource congregants for making sense of the events of their life cycle, including these moments in adoption.

Additionally, the minister should be aware and acknowledge the losses associated with these events when they occur. As Carrie Doehring suggests, a "psychic loss," like the hopes crushed by a failed adoption plan is very much a real loss for a waiting or adoptive family, as are the physical losses with failed and ruptured adoptions. Again, helping the church move through losses of all types through the normal course of preaching and worship can take the forms of both preparation and triage.

»   *Loss/grief for birthparents, extended families, and adoptees*

We could include birthparents in the above section on waiting, but it is important not to ignore birthparents, who wait with a particular kind of expectation. Instead of awaiting an addition, birthparents (and their extended families) await a loss. The times of waiting from knowledge of the pregnancy to making an adoption plan to the events of delivery and entrustment to the adoptive family are significant. While both birthfather and birthmother may experience difficult decisions and the psychological/emotional/spiritual weight of preparing for an adoption, the pastoral needs of birthmothers who carry and nurture the child(ren) to term will be especially acute. Birthparents will experience loss and probably, but not certainly, grief over that loss.

A very meaningful pastoral question to explore in this regard would be "What does it mean to prepare ourselves for a loss, knowing that the loss will be a blessing to others?" In this regard, the story of Hannah or Mary (who mirrors Hannah's story in the Gospel of Luke) would be particularly important. Pastors might even turn to the story of Jesus who, in the words of Philippians 2:7, "emptied himself" (*kenosis*) for the sake of others. In these characters, birthparents can find faithful examples through which they might identify, explore, and celebrate their decisions. A sermon or act of worship that makes the parallel between birthparents and Hannah, Mary, or Jesus could be an important part of their journey, inviting places of identification, exploration, and celebration. It could also help prospective adoptive parents as well as extended families see making an adoption plan from a new perspective.

Extended families of birthparents face loss as well. Extended families may feel as if they are losing grandchildren, nieces/nephews, and cousins. Some adjust well to this loss and encourage birthparents in their decisions; others do not and raise their objections. The pastoral care needs of extended families of birthparents within congregations should also be a priority for preaching and worship. In this case, communicating the Pauline theology of adoption as gift may be especially helpful. Finding ways to praise women like Moses' mother and Hannah for their courage to do what seemed best for their situations is a worthy goal for preaching and liturgical acts.

Adoptees can also experience multiple types of loss. Adoptees who grow up with closed adoptions (domestically or internationally, by choice or circumstance), may feel a significant loss with regard to their biological roots and identity. Accompanying that type of loss may be the sense of loss of one's culture of origin, particularly of those children adopted internationally and brought to the United States. Ministers should be sensitive that even as much as they might emphasize the gift language from the biblical witness as it concerns adoption, grief and loss may still linger concurrently with the feeling of gift. Making sense of gift and loss concurrently will be a complex process. Ministers will be careful in the language of preaching and worship to validate both, providing an environment that gives adoptees permission to be present with and explore their feelings. In this case, the stories of Moses and Genubath are helpful biblical narratives.

In all these cases, as outlined in chapter two, this is the pastoral work of "reaffirming personhood." Though birthparents, birth families, and adoptees may sense loss, it does not diminish their personhood before God or the community of faith. Ministers will be careful to keep this in mind and work toward liturgical environments that affirm individuals of their wholeness before God, despite the losses or fragmentation they may experience.

»   *New family bonds/networks*

While biological parents and extended families spend nine months establishing and nurturing bonds with their anticipated child, adoptive families do not get these opportunities, at least not in the same ways. Even if a waiting family has the privilege of getting to meet and know a birthmother from an early point in her pregnancy, they will not have the same experiences of establishing a relationship with the child *in utero* as a birthmother does.

In that light, whenever and however a child is placed with an adoptive family, that family must find new and meaningful ways to create the bonds of family. Extended families will need to establish new family networks as well. There are certainly basic physiological and emotional ways to do this. For instance, when my wife and I brought our daughter home at four days old without having previously established a relationship with her birthparents, we were instructed that one way we could establish our bonds and attachment with her could come through being the only ones who fed her or changed her diaper. While this was hard for some of our extended family to understand, in hindsight it played an invaluable role in developing trust and emotional closeness between our daughter and us.

Though I have given an example of establishing physiological and emotional bonds, ministers and congregations can play a key role in mediating the creation of family bonds and networks.[92] The idea of "entrustment" is a theme that can emerge in preaching and worship. Entrustment is a key word that emerges in several places in the New Testament in regard to how the faithful were given the precious message of salvation and now have the sacred responsibility to care for, preserve, and protect that message.[93] The parallels here are not difficult to draw: what once was not ours has been carefully considered and delivered over to us with sacred trust. That trust given assumes that not only will we do no harm to what has been given, but we will also provide the conditions for it to grow and thrive. Entrustment includes and values birth-parents as partners in the adoption triad (known or unknown), celebrating their trust that adoptive parents will provide a lifetime of care for children. The idea of entrustment is closely related to "stewardship" in the biblical context and outside it. I do not use the word stewardship here because even though the biblical idea of stewardship represents well the concept of entrustment, the word "stewardship" has become so connected to monetary giving in the context of congregations that I think it unhelpful in relation to adoption. Entrustment ceremonies, which I will outline later, can be performed by ministers in hospitals or in worship services, thus creating a rich and meaningful spiritual context for fostering bonds and family networks.

---

92 We might also consider this a "priestly" task. See Kenyatta Gilbert's discussion the priestly task of preaching in Kenyatta R. Gilbert, *The Journey and Promise of African American Preaching* (Minneapolis: Fortress Press, 2011).

93 See, for instance, Romans 6:17, 2 Corinthians 5:19, Galatians 2:7, 1 Timothy 6:20, Jude 1:3, among others.

Prophetic Tasks

Again, the lines between the pastoral and prophetic are not so distinct when it comes to preaching and worship. What is pastoral may also be considered prophetic, depending on the context and perspective of the minister, congregation, groups within a congregation and/or individual congregants. In chapter 2, I identify the prophetic as a kind of theologically reflective "talking back" to dominant, often uncritically received cultural (and religious) scripts that send us messages about what we are to say, think, do, or be. With this in mind, there are some specific tasks of preaching with adoption in view.

»   *Encourage and value adoption*

One of the primary ways ministers and congregations can "talk back" to dominant scripts in society at large is to encourage and value adoption in the language we use. As Jeanne Stevenson-Moessner observes, "Adoption is sometimes considered a joke. Kenneth Kaye remembers that he and his cousins 'would tease the younger ones by pretending to let slip the fact they were adopted. In reality, no one was; it was simply a way of saying, 'You're different; you'll never fit in.' We inherited the joke from our mothers, who have been recycling it on their baby sister for nearly 60 years.'"[94] Many of us may be able to identify this kind of playful talk in our families or playgrounds. Adoption often appears as a joke on commercials, television shows, and movies. It becomes a cheap punch line used to suggest that something has been hidden from a child; the resulting revelation will make sense of all her differences from her family and validate her feelings as an outsider.

Lingering inside adoption as joke is the idea of adoption as scandal, adoption as something for which guilt is necessary, or adoption as something that highlights difference and nullifies family. Because children may not know one or both of their birthparents, adoption may feel scandalous. Stevenson-Moessner reports that an "adopted

---

94 Jeanne Stevenson Moessner, "Womb-Love: The Practice and Theology of Adoption," *Christian Century* 118, no. 3 (2001): 10.

child felt treated differently by her teacher; the teacher made comments like: 'You think because you've gone through one experience in your life [the adoption], you've paid all your dues."[95] Other adoptive parents and children who have pronounced racial-ethnic or physiological differences from each other can be approached (often by complete strangers!) who will ask intrusive questions about the security of an adoptive relationship ("Aren't you worried that the birth family will try to take her back?"), countries of origin, or physiological features (hair color/type, skin color, facial/body features, etc.). These unsolicited conversations can be accompanied by unreflective comments about the nature of "real family." Undoubtedly these kinds of conversations happen often and can be unsettling to parents and children, undermining the significant work done to create family bonds.

In congregational worship, ministers can shape sermons and liturgical acts that press back on these negative, damaging messages. Ministers can intentionally craft language that celebrates families that come in all different shapes, sizes, forms, and configurations. As ministers outline the adopted status of all the people of God through Jesus Christ, we find that we acquire a family woven together out of every race, ethnicity, skin color, eye shape, hair type, etc. Adoption is not a joke or scandal; it is not guilt-inducing, nor is it something that highlights our differences in a negative way. Rather, adoption is the way God achieves God's purposes of salvation in and for the world. The way of God's salvation in the world is a model for how adoptive families are constructed and celebrated by the community of faith.

» *Shaping the language used in a community*

It may seem like "inside baseball" to some, but there are preferred ways to talk about the world of adoption. These choices in language are intended to stave off the stigma and shame attached to adoption in culture at-large. Variously called "adoption-friendly language" and "positive/negative language about adoption," such

---

95   Ibid.

changes in language are employed with regularity. Throughout this work we have already used many of these choices. For instance, "birthparent" or "biological mother/father" are used as opposed to "real parent" and "parent" over "adoptive parent."[96] The phrases "terminate parental rights" and "make an adoption plan" are used in place of "give up" and "give away" since those latter phrases place a negative emphasis on the actions of birthparents. Many say that a child "was adopted" rather than "is adopted" as a way of making adoption about the process of the child's placement in the past, rather than an enduring marker that defines a child for life. These are among the most important phrases.

Just as many ministers are careful about the language they use to refer to God, so too does the language surrounding adoption make a difference in preaching and worship. Language choices have the power to name the world, theologically speaking, and to shape the theological worldview of those gathered for worship. Adoption-friendly language is an act of liturgical inclusion, making sure that everyone in the adoption triad feels valued and there is nothing to hide.

It is important to carefully consider the normativity of bio-logical families in the language of preaching and worship as well. Jeanne Stevenson-Moessner tells a story about "Father Ron" and his sermon during a Wednesday mass.[97] Father Ron was devel-oping Colossians 1:15, which testifies that Jesus is "the image of the invisible God, the firstborn of all creation," and highlighted how children look like their parents, pointing to the physical re-semblances among the children and parents in the congregation that evening. Stevenson-Moessner says, "The point was profoundly simple: We know what God is like by looking at Jesus."[98] As Father Ron continued, he saw the agreement on the faces of a pair of girls who were sisters, one from India and one from Southeast Asia,

---

96 Though I have used "adoptive parent" throughout the course of this work as a matter of distinction.
97 Moessner, "Womb-Love: The Practice and Theology of Adoption," 10.
98 Ibid.

who happened to have Caucasian parents. Eventually, Father Ron realized the paradigm he was setting up as he surveyed his congregation. At that point, he acknowledged the families who had adopted children among the congregation and asked the children to raise their hands. "Now," Stevenson-Moessner observes, "the children were confronted with a choice: either hide their identity from the Catholic priest, or reveal an aspect of themselves that some children consider personal or private. Hands went up at half-mast."[99] The language we use in preaching and worship, even as we make "profoundly simple" theological observations, makes a difference to how those gathered for worship construct their worlds and see themselves.

» *Combatting "adoption chic" and the commodification of children*

A final prophetic task is to combat what I call "adoption chic" and the commodification of children through adoption. This idea is two-pronged; the first being the "cool factor" of entering the adoption process, particularly the intercountry adoption process. We have certainly seen celebrities like Angelina Jolie, Madonna, and Katherine Heigl among others adopt from the African continent and Southeast Asia. To some extent these celebrities have set a precedent, as with fashion, on ways to grow a family which often mask the realities associated with intercountry adoption. As a result, it is not uncommon to hear people make statements about how "cool it would be to adopt from X country" and about "how cute *those* babies are," which strikes me not only as racist (the novelty of the "exotic" brown baby with the white parents has twinges of racism and colonialism, in my opinion), but also naïve about the realities of intercountry adoption. I should be clear that I do not want to be dismissive of anyone's motivations to adopt, but I am wary about this phenomenon.

Likewise, I once heard a story relayed from an attendee at a large Evangelical congregation about how a young women's group

---

99 Ibid.

had gotten the international adoption bug. Young (white) women with biological children who gathered regularly were seemingly entering into a string of adoptions. The person who relayed this story to me described the pressure the group exerted on its members to adopt a child from another country and how strange the mentality of the group felt. A 2013 article from news outlet *Mother Jones* highlights the "adoption fever" of some Evangelicals and the harmful results of that fever, including failed and ruptured adoptions as well as severe emotional and psychological problems on the part of adopted children stemming from lack of oversight in the adoption process and poor parenting.[100]

Associated with "adoption chic" is the commodification of child acquisition. Unfortunately, celebrity adoptions and upwardly mobile, affluent Americans interested in adoption produce the side effects of a mentality of commodification by many parties. Diplomats, international and domestic agencies and their liaisons, caretakers, and prospective parents get caught in a web where children are simply seen as commodities. Birthparents become easy targets, as do prospective families whose emotional desires for children make them easy prey. Again, there are always fees associated with adoptions and I must confess, there were times when I wrote a large check feeling as if I was empowered to "buy" the opportunity for a child. While I was not taken advantage of, some are. What I am describing, however, is a pervasive culture that imagines children as goods to be purchased, even when the processes of those adoptions are completely above board (and they are not always above board).[101]

---

100 Kathryn Joyce, "Orphan Fever: The Evangelical Movement's Adoption Obsession," http://www.motherjones.com/politics/2013/04/christian-evangelical-adoption-liberia. See also Brandon T. Maxwell, "'Christian' Americanity and the New Gospel of Adoption," http://theparkinglotblog.com/2013/06/10/christian-americanity-the-new-gospel-of-adoption/.

101 For the convergence of commodification and Evangelicalism, see Jen Hatmaker, "Examining Adoption Ethics: Part One," http://jenhatmaker.com/blog/2013/05/14/examining-adoption-ethics-part-one.

The ways that preaching and worship touch this problem should be direct. Ministers can portray the realities of adoption and parenthood versus the fragments we encounter in our glimpses of celebrity culture, or encourage prospective adoptive parents to consult those who have adopted, lifting up those who have had successes and supporting those who have had difficulties. In preaching, ministers can bring to light the examples of harmful adoption services. Ministers can also pray and preach in specific ways against those that would do harm to the lives of children. This is truly in the tradition of the biblical prophets, as we highlighted in the previous chapter. Extending justice and care to the orphan means treating them not as if they are objects to be collected, bought, and sold but rather as those who receive the love and justice of God's care.

PLANS FOR PREACHING AND WORSHIP

We have traced some large-scale, adoption-specific tasks for preaching and worship. As discussed above, some of these tasks will occur in the normal course of preaching and planning worship. But how does the minister plan preaching and worship in a strategic manner to intentionally engage these tasks when they might not naturally occur in the course of congregational life?

Since adoption is rooted in the biblical witness in some significant and overwhelmingly positive ways, and preaching and worship take their cues from the pulse of the biblical story, there is no reason to avoid the realities of adoption in public worship. One option might be to utilize a topical preaching/worship series, planning a course of worship services that center around issues of family and perhaps, difficult or rarely addressed family issues. This could include the two main topics in this work, but also issues like abuse within the family, divorce, blended families, marriage enrichment, singleness and dating, loss of family members, etc. In a topical series, ministers can offer the biblical witness in ways that are contextually appropriate for their congregations, picking and choosing the texts that are most helpful.

Many mainline denominational ministers use the Revised Common Lectionary (hereafter referred to as "RCL") as the textual basis for weekly preaching and worship planning. The RCL provides some encouragement for working with the characters and stories we have mentioned. In this way, if there is some trepidation about addressing the topic of adoption, the minister will have multiple chances to address it at some point in the three-year lectionary cycle as possibilities occur in years A, B, and C.

- Abram and Eliezer's story in Genesis 15 occurs in Year C, on both the 2nd Sunday after Lent and Proper 14, giving ministers two opportunities to address this text.
- Moses' story in Exodus 1:8-2:10 occurs in Year A, Proper 16.
- Hannah and Samuel's story in 1 Samuel 1:4-20 occurs in Year B, Proper 28. Hannah's song is included in Years A, B, and C on the celebration of the Visitation of Mary, since it parallels Mary's Magnificat.
- Obed and Naomi's in Ruth 3:1-5; 4:13-17 occurs in Year B, Proper 27.
- A portion of Esther's story, Esther 7:1-6, 9-10; 9:20-22 occurs in Year B, Proper 21. Even though this is a small selection from Esther that does not include her birth/adoption narrative, this is easily enough included in telling Esther and Mordecai's story.
- Psalm 68:1-10, 32-35 occurs in Year A, Seventh Sunday of Easter
- Psalm 82 occurs in Year C on Propers 10 and 15
- Isaiah 1:1, 10-20 occurs in Year C, Proper 14 and 1:10-28 occurs in Year C on Proper 26.
- Psalm 146 occurs in Year B on Propers 18, 26, and 27 and in Year C on Propers 5 and 21. Psalm 146:5-10 occurs in Year A on the Third Sunday of Advent.

- Romans 8:12-17 occurs in Year B, Trinity Sunday; 8:12-25 occurs in Year A, Proper 11; 8:14-17 occurs in Year C, Day of Pentecost; 8:22-27 occurs in Year B, Day of Pentecost; Romans 9:1-5 occurs in Year A, Proper 13.

- Galatians 4:4-7 occurs in Year A, B, and C on the Feast of the Holy Name of Jesus and in Year B, First Sunday after Christmas Day.

- Ephesians 1:3-14 occurs in Years A, B, and C on the Second Sunday after Christmas Day and in Year B, Proper 10.

- James 1:17-27 occurs in Year B, Proper 17.

Of course, not all these characters and passages make an appearance in the RCL. Ephraim and Manasseh's story in Genesis 47, Jephthah's story in Judges 11, and Genubath in 1 Kings 11 are all excluded from the RCL cycles. The texts from Deuteronomy, Job, Proverbs, Jeremiah, Ezekiel, Hosea, Zechariah, and Malachi are omitted, as well as some of the Psalms. Those who are familiar with the RCL know it is an imperfect collection, even as it sweeps broadly across both testaments.

Given the biblical texts and stories we might want to explore as it relates to adoption, Luther Seminary's "narrative lectionary" provides another helpful option, or more precisely, a helpful direction for a series or episodes of preaching. The narrative lectionary "is a four-year cycle of readings. On the Sundays from September through May each year the texts follow the sweep of the biblical story, from Creation through the early Christian church. The texts show the breadth and variety of voices within Scripture. They invite people to hear the stories of Abraham and Sarah, Moses and the prophets, Jesus, and Paul. Listening to the many different voices within Scripture enriches preaching and the life of faith."[102] The intention is to hear the biblical witness as a wide, continuous narrative, rather than the often choppy, discontinuous nature of the RCL. Included here are the stories of Ruth and Naomi (a partial

---

102 "Narrative Lectionary FAQ," http://www.workingpreacher.org/narrative_faqs.aspx.

offering from chapter 1) and Hannah and Samuel. Though there are only two selections included here, the impulse behind the narrative lectionary is of merit: there is a large biblical narrative to be told. A minister could also put together a series of worship services entitled something like "God's Adoption Story," exploring the ways that the biblical witness employs adoption and orphan care.

Since some of these stories leave details to be desired and since none of them are complete, the art of *midrash* may be appropriate here. Midrash is a Jewish style of interpretation that seeks to provide commentary on scripture. In contemporary context with homiletic and liturgical application, midrash is a type of commentary on the scriptures that imaginatively fills in the gaps and missing details in the biblical texts. In this case, preaching and worship can seek to faithfully explore the gaps in the biblical stories. What details are missing in the stories and passages that relate to adoption and orphan care? What thoughts and feelings accompany the characters in the story or writers like the Psalmist and Paul? How do the characters thrive, survive, or suffer because of what has happened in their lives? Engaging in midrash for these passages provides the opportunity for the kind of narrative space described in the previous chapter. This allows worshippers to walk around in the shoes of the biblical character, using their spiritual, emotional, and psychological space for their own reflection. In practice the sermon could take the form of a dramatic first-person monologue from the perspective of one of the characters in or associated with the biblical text. Or there may be a dramatic rendering of the story at some point in the worship service that takes the form of midrash, with the preacher executing midrashic interpretation during the course of the sermon.

Up to this point, I have assumed that many congregations will follow the liturgical year with regard to preaching and worship. The liturgical year provides a broader context for tracing the biblical story. But the liturgical year does not always capture every date that a congregation deems important for its life together. For instance, in my congregation we observe "Worship in Pink" once a year to honor and remember those who have battled breast cancer. Other congregations will observe Mother's or Father's Day or patriotic days that fall close to a Sunday.

While this is not part of the liturgical year, CAFO sponsors "Orphan Sunday" on the first Sunday in November. For congregations interested in raising awareness, promoting faithful action, and celebrating the adoption triad, this might be a possible addition. Regarding the date and the name, this need not be the tradition of every church. A congregation might decide to celebrate "Forever Family Sunday," picking a date meaningful to a family or families within the congregation around the anniversary of an adoption finalization or the day a family member came home (variously known as "Family Days" or "Gotcha Days"). With the same purposes, a congregation could celebrate in worship the bonds of adoptive families, raise awareness, and encourage further action. Worship on that day could include the testimony of those who have positively experienced adoption from various perspectives, prayer for waiting families, blessing of adoptive families, entrustment ceremonies, or other appropriate ideas.

Liturgical Actions

With regard to the worship service and acts of worship beyond preaching, ministers will want to make available a number of ways for adoptive families to mark this time in the life cycle through ritual. Susan White notes that "the service of thanksgiving for the birth or adoption of a child is a way of bringing before God the hopes, desires, and (perhaps) anxieties of parents for their child; of expressing the joy at new beginnings; and of giving voice to the Christian community's prayers for the family."[103] If the congregation has been a community of care for the family throughout the adoption process, a service of thanksgiving can be a special time of celebration and a changing commitment to play a role in the

---

103 Susan J. White, *Foundations of Christian Worship*, 1st U.S. ed. (Louisville, KY: Westminster John Knox Press, 2006), 136.

child's growth. Older children who are new to a congregational community may find a broader network of support, inclusion, and integration through this kind of service. Though I do not come from a tradition that baptizes infants, some families will want to bring together the thanksgiving for adoption and a service of baptism (or, in my case, dedication). Some denominational worship books include services of thanksgiving for adoptions. Examples and references to services of thanksgiving are provided in the in the Appendix.

In congregations where birthparents and birth families are present and have been open in their decision to make an adoption plan and have a high level of comfort, a minister might plan a service of prayer and blessing for birthparents and birth families (with full permission and cooperation from birthparents and birth families, of course). This could be a kind of preparatory service of prayer and blessing, as birthparents prepare to finalize an adoption plan and entrust a child to an adoptive family. Or this kind of service could be a way to offer blessing as the birth family transitions into a different life phase of its life cycle. This has the potential to move birth families out of the shadows, providing them with the blessing of the Christian community, rather than the guilt and shame they might feel.

Entrustment ceremonies will likely be rarer in the experience of the minister, but as open adoptions continue to rise in the U.S., the entrustment ceremony may continue to become more necessary for the minister's liturgical repertoire. While an entrustment service could be used in a number of different scenarios, it will most likely be used in conjunction with a domestic, open infant adoption. In this case, the entrustment ceremony will not be celebrated in a church (though there is no reason it could not be), but in a hospital chapel with any birth family members, adoptive family members, social workers, hospital chaplain/staff, and/or ministers as the birth family and adoptive family agree to involve. Preparation and planning will be key for the adoptive family and the presiding minister. The idea of an entrustment service is to ritualize what can otherwise be an awkward transition of a child from birth family to adoptive family. This gives an open adoption firm footing in blessing, prayer, and as the name of the service suggests, trust given from birth family to adoptive family. Again, an example of an entrustment service is included in the Appendix.

Other types of services may arise given the different contours adoption takes in each new context. Ruth Duck helps us think about creating new pastoral liturgies for these changing life situations by giving a basic outline of new pastoral liturgies:

-   A brief statement of the human situation that led to this liturgy, perhaps through a personal statement, litany of remembrance, or reading [a statement of purpose]
-   Some witness to God's presence with us in this situation through Scripture, sermon, testimonies about the movement from pain or anger to faith and hope, or assurance of the community's support
-   A prayer or ritual act that helps persons move into the future with hope and commitment through laying on of hands for healing or commissioning, presenting the gift of a small green plant as a symbol of growing life, burning or tossing of symbols of letting go, or making personal expressions of intention
-   Sending forth with a charge based on intentions expressed and a blessing naming God's presence in all we do

"Such liturgies," Duck observes, "express the love of the community and of God in every situation in life."[104]

The church's preaching and worship life can be especially life-giving as adoption continues to emerge in the public eye. Rather than silence or avoidance, ministers who do the work of preaching and planning/leading worship with an eye toward adoption give a strong theological lens to their congregations, helping them frame adoption with grace and truth.

---

104 Ruth C. Duck, *Worship for the Whole People of God: Vital Worship for the 21st Century* (Louisville, KY: Westminster John Knox Press, 2013), 230.

Appendix

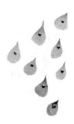

In this short appendix, I offer some selected resources for preaching and worship, including two brief portions of sermons and various types of resources for public worship.

Sermon Portion #1

This portion of a sermon on James 5:13-20 attempted to "break the silence" about reproductive difficulty, linking together James' instructions about suffering with the directive to pray, even when prayer itself is difficult.

In the Spring of 2006, my wife and I decided that we would try to enlarge our family with children. Like many young professional couples, we had delayed that process, attending graduate school and struggling to pay off student debt and replace cars that had died and all the while thinking that we would be able to have children on our schedule and at will. That wasn't to be the case. Despite our best efforts and the efforts of medical intervention, and through many cycles of hope and despair, we were denied. Then as we decided to pursue adoption, we went through 2 more years of waiting and more cycles of hope and despair. Most of you obviously know the curly-haired, smiling face of a blessing that ends that story, but the in-between times were simply awful and lonely. Those times were full of doubt, pain, and angry prayers to God.

I filled many pages of a prayer journal with words asking where God was and what God might be up to. I laid awake at night echoing the words of the Psalmist, "How long, O Lord, how long?" I hurled up prayers as the ceiling fan spun round and round, almost as if that fan was chopping up those prayers like a blender and hurling them into the far reaches of time and space, eluding even God's abilities to grab them and put them back together.

You've stared at that ceiling fan, haven't you? With a dull, nagging ache in the pit of your stomach about what's missing in your life, agonizing over a job lost, a relationship with a friend or spouse or parent or relative broken, a life taken too soon, a body that will not do what it's designed to do, an addiction that you cannot keep at bay, an emotional or psychological wound that will not heal, a situation that looks like a dead end. You've laid awake at night and stared at that same ceiling fan, haven't you?

SERMON PORTION #2

This portion of a sermon on Romans 8:22-27 was the final sermon I preached in my ministry at Central Christian Church (Disciples of Christ) in Springfield, TN. This is a church that, though small in number, had an extraordinary representation of adoption stories.

We live in a world where things are not right. We stand in this world as church with a profound sense that God's work is not yet done. In fact, we see right in front of us, as Paul says to the church at Rome, "the whole creation groaning in labor pains." When we jump into this section of Romans, we're jumping into a larger conversation about salvation. And here, even though Paul affirms the existence of the terrible—the groaning of creation and the suffering of both earth and humanity, he also tells us resolutely: God has done something in this world right here and now. And not just that. Paul anticipates that God will do more.

God has done something about the present conditions, the suffering of this world. Having previously been a key player in the suffering problem, Paul knew the reality of God having acted decisively through Jesus. After his Damascus Road encounter with the Risen Christ, Paul was assured that God had brought the promise of redemption through Jesus. Paul knew that salvation was God's love for all people, regardless of their past or their present.

And so like Paul, we too live into the confidence of God's salvation. Paul talks about the promise of God's salvation right now and compares it to adoption – an adoption that is simultaneously complete and not yet fully accomplished.

Luckily adoption is something this church knows about in different ways. In different ways, we know about being brought into the family of God; we know the waiting and work it takes to be signed and sealed by the judge. Paul hints to us that salvation is not just forgiveness of sins, it's not simply a heavenly reward. Instead, part of the beauty of our salvation is that in Christ we enter into a new kind of family. Through Christ we live into reordered relationships between God and humanity—we participate fully in that reordering.

Part of why the image of "family" is so strong in this congregation and many others like ours is that in Christ we find new relationships that bring us toward healing and wholeness right here and right now. In the midst of the suffering of the world and our own personal suffering, we can rejoice because we know that God has seen fit to bring us into God's household with one another.

Still, we do not rest in that knowledge because we know that the world is not yet what it shall be. We know our salvation here and now, but we also sit in expectation of God's bringing all things to completion. We believe in the promise Paul describes – that God isn't finished with us or with this world.

PASTORAL PRAYERS FROM MOTHER'S AND FATHER'S DAYS

The following two prayers, similar in format, were written for use during the Pastoral Prayer on Mother's Day and Father's Day, respectively. In them I seek to honor those who have experienced reproductive difficulty as well as members of the adoption triad.

Loving God,
You approach us with great care. Like a mother hen you gather us under your wings and you hold us close. We celebrate this morning the ways that you love us.

You are slow to anger, abounding in steadfast love.

You protect us from ourselves and other forces that would cause us harm.

You desire no one to turn away from you – so much so that you sent Jesus Christ to show us the depths of your love.

In Jesus we find the fullness of your love.

Even so, God there are people and places that seem distant from your love, even though you are never beyond our reach.

We pray for the sick, who need your healing touch.

We pray for those at war, that they may find your peace.

We pray for those who are lonely and confused, that they may find the comfort of your presence.

We pray for those who do not know where they will sleep tonight, that they may find shelter through those who love you.

We pray for those who mourn, that they might know, through their grief, the hope of resurrection.

We pray for those who do not know you. Give us the courage to share our deep knowledge of your love.

And on this day, we call Mother's Day we pray especially for mothers.

We are thankful for the presence of loving mothers in our lives, both living and those who await the Resurrection. Help mothers and grandmothers to continue to embody the love we see in your motherly image, O God.

We pray for those who have been abused by mothers and for those mothers who perpetrate abuse. Bring them a full measure of your healing and restoration, O God.

We pray for mothers who are unsure of how they will feed their children today, of how they will pay their bills. Grant to them the resources to care for their families and help us to be a part of that provision.

We pray for single mothers, especially those who have little support for the stressful job of being a parent. Surround them with people who can make their lives easier.

We pray for birthmothers who have made hard decisions, but who have given families joy through their courage. Let them know how they have blessed others through their decisions.

We pray for those who serve as mothers for others despite not having given birth to the children they care for: for aunts and cousins and close family friends. Rain down your blessings on them for being a loving presence.

We also pray this morning for those who are, or were, for whatever reason, unable to have children. For those whose bodies have betrayed them, for those who wait in what seems to be in endless cycles of hope and despair, and for those whose circumstances deny them. Comfort them in their loss and grief for this indeed is a difficult day for them.

All of this we pray in the name of Jesus, who taught us to pray…

Loving God,

Almost without thought, we often address you as Father. We celebrate this morning the ways that your love for us typifies what we hope for and need in fathers.

You teach and guide us and give us boundaries, even as you show us the possibilities for our lives.

You protect us from ourselves and other forces that would cause us harm.

You desire no one to turn away from you—so much so that you sent Jesus Christ to show us the depths of your love.

In Jesus we find the fullness of your love.

Even so, God there are people and places that seem distant from your love, even though you are never beyond our reach.

We pray for the sick, who need your healing touch.

We pray for those at war, that they may find your peace.

We pray for those who are lonely and confused, that they may find the comfort of your presence.

We pray for those who do not know where they will sleep tonight, that they may find shelter   through those who love you.

We pray for those who mourn, that they might know, through their grief, the hope of resurrection.

And on this day, we call Father's Day we pray for fathers.

We are thankful for the presence of loving fathers in our lives. Help fathers and grandfathers to continue to embody the love we see in your fatherly image, O God.

We pray for those who have recently lost fathers and grandfathers, and those who sit on the precipice of loss. Bring to mind the life lessons learned and warm memories they have shared.

We pray for those who have been abused by fathers and for those fathers who perpetrate abuse against their children and spouses. Bring them a full measure of your healing and restoration, O God.

We pray for fathers who are unsure of how they will provide for their children today, of how they will pay their bills. Grant to them the resources to care for their families.

We pray for single fathers who have little support for the stressful job of being a parent. Surround them with people who can make their lives easier.

We also pray this morning for those who are, for whatever reason, unable to have children. For those whose bodies have betrayed them, for those whose circumstances deny them. Comfort them in their loss and grief for this indeed is a difficult day for them.

All of this we pray in the name of Jesus, who taught us to pray…

1. AN ENTRUSTMENT CEREMONY

The following is an outline for an Entrustment Ceremony writ-ten by Becky Baile Crouse.[105]*As discussed previously, this most likely might be performed with an open, domestic infant adoption within the hospital setting.*

- Opening words, with a reading from Psalm 139:13-16
- A short opening reminding those gathered of God's care for children

» **Praise and Presentation**

- Praising God for the child, whose transitions into a different stage of life as well as thanksgiving for the birth family. Crouse briefly narrates the story of Moses and the network of care surrounding his birth and then names the ritual as one of entrustment and the forging of sacred, spiritual bonds.
- [If there is some question about who will hold the child during the service, the adoptive parents may hold the child for the entire service or the birthparents may hand the child over to the adoptive parents at this point.]
- Family sharing
- An opportunity for anyone present to speak or a moment of silence

» **Musical sharing**

- Crouse suggests that simple songs from the Christian tradition about children might be used.

» **Words of Commitment**

- Crouse offers words of pledge, shared by both birth family and adoptive family, with an invited response.

---

105 Becky Baile Crouse, "An Entrustment Service for Families Participating in Open Adoption," *Chaplaincy Today* 23, no. 1 (2007).

» **Blessing**

– The minister pronounces a blessing over the child.

» **Prayer and Benediction**

– The minister prays for all gathered in ways appropriate to their roles beyond this moment then blesses those who are gathered.

THANKSGIVING AND BLESSING OF ADOPTION

The following is an outline of a service for the blessing of an adoption written by Henry T. Close.[106]

– The Meaning of Adoption
– A statement of purpose and the significance of adoption
– Prayer
– Acceptance of Responsibility

Close describes this ceremony as one where older siblings were present and it was important for the older siblings to be able to pledge their lives as siblings to the new infant child, as well as the parents to reaffirm their responsibility to the older children. If the ceremony took place in a congregational setting, it would be most appropriate to involve the congregation in pledging their responsibility as well.

» **An Allegory on Being a Family**

– This is a meditation or, in the context of weekly worship, could be a sermon.

» **The Exchange of Gifts**

– Again, with the older siblings present, it was important to allow them an opportunity to give to the new sibling.

---

106 Henry T. Close, "An Adoption Ceremony," *Journal of Pastoral Care* 47, no. 4 (1993).

The parents gave gifts to the older siblings as well. Again, if the ceremony were to take place within a congregational setting, it would be appropriate for a representative of the congregation (or the children of the congregation) to give all the children gifts of some kind.
- The Lord's Prayer
- Declaration

Many denominational worship books now include services of thanksgiving and celebration for an adoption. Those that do not have specific services for adoption may have services for children that have recently been born. Those services may have interchangeable parts, substitutions for adoption, or can often easily be adapted to suitably address adoption. For instance, my tradition's worship book, Chalice Worship, *offers a service of blessing for children which could be adapted for the purposes of celebrating an adoption. Since there are a number of services available, and this resource is meant to be suggestive rather than exhaustive, I will outline below the service from the* United Methodist Book of Worship, *which is commendable even in its simplicity. This service is shorter than the one above, and is meant for use within a weekly service of worship. Elements of both services could be combined, depending on context. For instance, I would suggest combining the "Acceptance of Responsibility" from the service above (or what I would call "Covenant-Making") with the service below.*

» **Presentation and Call to Thanksgiving**
- This act can be done as an act of Response to the Word or at another place that is appropriate. In the presentation, parents and children come forward and the minister states the purpose of this act of worship, inviting the congregation to join the family in welcome, celebration, and thanksgiving.

»   **Prayer of Thanksgiving and Intercession**

–   The prayer references God's adoption of humanity, gives
     thanks for the child, and asks for blessings on the family.

»   **Song of Response and Blessing**

–   Suitable songs are suggested for this moment and a short
     blessing can be pronounced on the family.

The Calvin Institute of Christian Worship also provides commendable sample services for the following: Receiving Adopted
Children, Baptism of Adopted Children, An Entrustment Ceremony, and Music/Songs for these events. See http://worship.
calvin.edu/resources/resource-library/resources-for-adoption-bap-
tism-services/

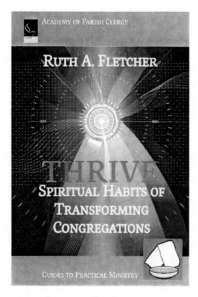
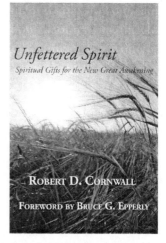

More from Energion Publications

CPSIA information can be obtained
at www.ICGtesting.com
Printed in the USA
LVOW11s0029180418
573737LV00001B/8/P